GERD

LICENSE, DISCLAIMER OF LIABILITY, AND LIMITED WARRANTY

GERD

Living With Acid Reflux Disease

David A. Olle

MERCURY LEARNING AND INFORMATION

Dulles, Virginia
Boston, Massachusetts
New Delhi

Publisher: David Pallai
MERCURY LEARNING AND INFORMATION
22841 Quicksilver Drive
Dulles, VA 20166
info@merclearning.com
www.merclearning.com
(800) 232-0223

This book is printed on acid-free paper.

David A. Olle. *GERD: Living With Acid Reflux Disease.*
ISBN: 978-1-942270-05-8

The publisher recognizes and respects all marks used by companies, manufacturers, and developers as a means to distinguish their products. All brand names and product names mentioned in this book are trademarks or service marks of their respective companies. Any omission or misuse (of any kind) of service marks or trademarks, etc. is not an attempt to infringe on the property of others.

Library of Congress Control Number: 2015902724
151617 3 2 1   Printed in the United States of America

Our titles are available for adoption, license, or bulk purchase by institutions, corporations, etc. For additional information, please contact the Customer Service Dept. at (800)232-0223(toll free).

All of our titles are available in digital format at authorcloudware.com and other digital vendors. Companion disc files for this title are available by contacting info@merclearning.com. The sole obligation of MERCURY LEARNING AND INFORMATION to the purchaser is to replace the disc, based on defective materials or faulty workmanship, but not based on the operation or functionality of the product.

Contents

PART FOUR Diagnosing and Treating GERD

CHAPTER 10 *Diagnosing GERD*

CHAPTER 11 *GERD Medications*

CHAPTER 12 *Surgical Procedures*

Acknowledgments

This book would not have been possible without the support and encouragement of the staff at Mercury Learning and Information, particularly David Pallai, publisher and founder, and Jennifer Blaney, project manager. The copy editor, Linda Alila, gave many suggestions and comments that helped to bring the manuscript to final form. I am especially thankful to my wife and daughters who have shown patience and understanding during this undertaking.

Introduction

Heartburn or acid reflux is a very common condition that is usually self-treated. Although usually considered to be benign, the condition can advance to more serious complications, when it is known as gastroesophageal reflux disease or GERD, the focus of this book.

This book is a comprehensive discussion of GERD for the general reader, and provides updates on many recent developments in the field. As background material, the book discusses basic terms followed by digestive tract anatomy as it relates to GERD. The common symptoms and the broad range of GERD complications are then discussed.

Usually the physician recommends lifestyle modifications as a first step in treating GERD. Changes in lifestyle allow the patient to take charge of his or her own treatment and can have benefits in addition to alleviating GERD. The book discusses the types of modifications and their effectiveness in alleviating GERD.

Many advances in medications to treat GERD have taken place, and some medications previously available only by prescription can now be obtained over-the-counter. The effectiveness, limitations, and potential side effects of the medications are clearly stated.

When lifestyle modifications or medications do not alleviate GERD, surgery is the last resort. Major advances in surgical procedures have taken place, particularly in the area of minimally invasive surgery. The newer procedures can involve less risk than conventional surgery, and patients can experience a quicker recovery with fewer complications.

I hope this book is informative and educational for you. Companion files (figures and related health files) for this title are available by contacting info@merclearning.com.

David A. Olle, MS
Guilford, VT

ulcer
eat
tissue medicine
digestion body
pain esophagu
human pepti
acid stomacl
endoscopy
sphincter ache physiolog
gastric duodenum biopsy
ttack organ health intestine
sorder reflux system abdomen
care medical disease anatomy
ancer gastrointestional
lness healthcare digest
cardia pylorus
healthy

PART ONE

Introduction to GERD: Definitions and Prevalence

In Part One, we introduce basic definitions relating to gastroesophageal reflux disease, and discuss the occurrence of GERD in the general population.

CHAPTER 1
What is GERD?

CHAPTER 2
How Prevalent is GERD?

What is GERD?

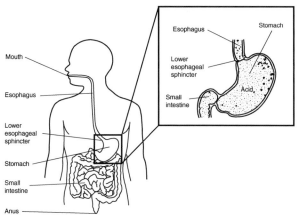

◄ **FIGURE 1.1**

Schematic drawing of digestive tract, with close-up of organs associated with GERD

SOURCE: National Digestive Diseases Information Clearinghouse (NDDIC)

1. What is gastroesophageal reflux (GER)?

Occasional GER is very common and may cause temporary discomfort such as heartburn or acid regurgitation.

Gastroesophageal reflux (GER), also known as **acid** reflux or **acid regurgitation**, occurs when stomach contents flow back up into the esophagus (NDDIC 2013).

2. What is gastroesophageal reflux disease (GERD)?

The presence of GERD is often defined as the occurrence of at least two reflux symptoms per week.

Gastroesophageal reflux disease (GERD) is a more serious, chronic—or long lasting—form of GER that includes symptoms and/or complications that affect the well-being of the person (Katz 2013).

3. What is acid reflux?

The stomach contents that flow back into the esophagus are commonly known as **acid reflux**, recognizing that the primary injurious component is hydrochloric acid, secreted by stomach glands. The main focus of GERD medical treatments is to prevent acid from being secreted into the stomach, or to neutralize stomach acid. The stomach contents that are refluxed, however, also consist of digestive enzymes, mucin, and partially digested food. These components are known as **non-acid reflux**, and may contribute to the detrimental effect of reflux (Hirschowitz 1999). The components of reflux in its entirety are known as refluxate. Non-acid reflux is discussed in Question 39.

4. What is a symptom?

A **symptom** is a departure from normal function or feeling that is noticed by a patient, indicating the presence of disease or abnormality. A symptom is subjective and cannot be measured directly.

DEFINITION

How Prevalent is GERD?

ulcer
eat
tissue medicine
digestion body
pain esophagus
human peptic
acid stomach
stric ache physiology
k organ health duodenum biopsy
reflux system abdomen
medical disease anatomy
gastrointestinal
dia healthcare digest
pylorus

5. What is prevalence?

Prevalence is the percentage of the population having a condition at a specific point in time or during a given period, such as three months.

DEFINITION

6. What is the overall prevalence of GERD?

Reviews of large research studies have indicated that about 10–20% of the US population experience symptoms of GERD at least weekly (Dent 2005). A recent review (2012) showed the prevalence of GERD to be around 18–27% in North America (El-Serag 2013). As mentioned, GER is more common. A typical study showed that around 45% of the population reported at least one reflux symptom over the past 3 months (Camilleri 2005), while another study found that up to 60% experienced symptoms at some time during the year.

For an excellent discussion of the epidemiology and risk factors associated with GERD, download the following article from the journal **Gut**:

NOTE

http://gut.bmj.com/content/54/5/710.full

7. Is there a sex difference in GERD prevalence?

Women may be more likely than men to develop GERD. Estrogens may play a role in increased GERD in women. Women receiving estrogen either naturally through menstrual cycles or by post-menopausal hormone therapy experience more GERD symptoms than pre- or postmenopausal women (Nilsson 2003). Pregnant women are more susceptible to GERD due to decreased LES pressures (explained in Chapter 2) (Jacobson 2008). The Federal Agency for Healthcare Research and Quality prepared a statistical brief stating that women accounted for 62% of all hospitalizations for GERD in 2005 (Zhao 2007). However, other studies did not show a significant association between sex and GERD (Dent 2005).

8. Does GERD affect people of all ages?

GERD can occur in people of all age groups from infants to elderly. GERD is most often diagnosed in individuals between the ages of 45 and 64 (about 50% of cases). Adults 65 and older have a lower prevalence of GERD symptoms (Ricci 2003). Children and infants have recently shown an increase in diagnosis of GERD.

To view an introductory video on GERD, visit:

https://www.youtube.com/watch?v=TdK0jRFpWPQ

References

CHAPTER 1

1   Hirschowitz, Basil. "Pepsin and the Esophagus." *Yale Journal of Biology and Medicine 72*, nos. 2–3 (1999): 133–143.

2   Katz, Philip O., Lauren B. Gerson, and Marcelo F. Vela. "Guidelines for the Diagnosis and Management of Gastroesophageal Reflux Disease." *American Journal of Gastroenterology*, vol. 108 (2013): 308–328.

3   National Digestive Diseases Information Clearinghouse. "Gastroesophageal Reflux (GER) and Gastroesophageal Reflux Disease (GERD) in Adults." NIH Publication No. 13–0882, Washington DC, 2013. http://www.niddk.nih.gov/health-information/health-topics/digestive-diseases/ger-and-gerd-in-adults/Documents/gerd_508.pdf

CHAPTER 2

4   Camilleri, Michael. "Prevalence and Socioeconomic Impact of Upper Gastrointestinal Disorders in the United States: Results of the US Upper Gastrointestinal Study." *Clinical Gastroenterology and Hepatology 3*, no. 6 (2005): 543–552.

5   Dent John, Hashem El-Sarag, Mari-Ann Wallander, and Saga Johansson. "Epidemiology of Gastro-oesophageal Reflux Disease: A Systematic Review." *Gut* 54, no. 5 (2005): 710–717.

6   El-Serag, Hashem, Stephen Sweet, Christopher Winchester, and John Dent. "Update on the Epidemiology of Gastro-oesophageal Reflux Disease: A Systematic Review." *Gut* 63, no. 6 (2014):871-880.

7   Jacobson, Brian C., Beverly Moy, Graham A. Colditz, and Charles S. Fuchs. "Postmenopausal hormone use and symptoms of gastroesophageal reflux." *Archives of Internal Medicine* 168, no. 16 (2008): 1798-1804.

8   Nilsson, Magnus, Roar Johnsen, Weimin Ye, Kristian Hveem, and Jesper Lagergren. "Obesity and Estrogen as Risk Factors for Gastroesophageal Reflux Symptoms." *Journal of the American Medical Association* 290, no. 1 (2003): 66-72.

9   Ricci Judith A., Luella Engelhart, Sheldon Sloan, and Carol Leotta. "Age differences in the Epidemiology and Treatment of GERD-Related Symptoms." Poster at International Society For Pharmacoeconomics and Outcomes Research (ISPOR) 8th Annual International Meeting, Arlington, VA, May 18–21, 2003.

10 Zhao, Yafu, and William Encinosa. "Gastroesophageal Reflux Disease (GERD) Hospitalizations in 1998 and 2005." Healthcare Cost and Utilization Project, Statistical Brief #44 (2008), http://www.hcup-us.ahrq.gov/reports/statbriefs/sb44.jsp

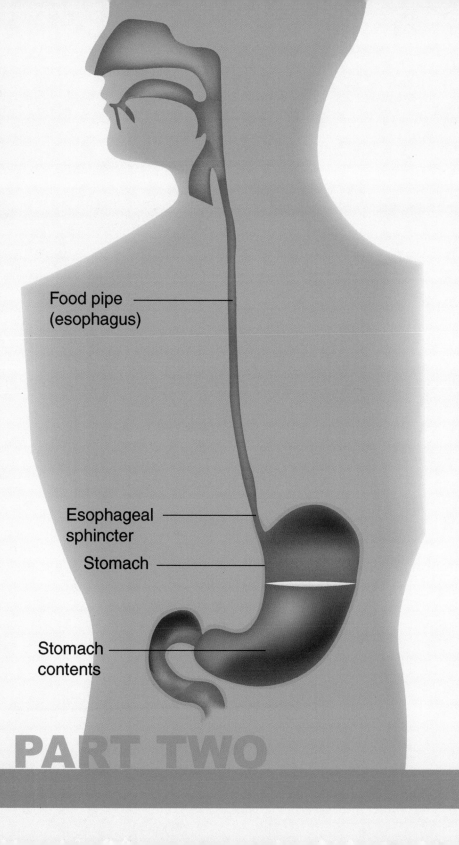

Food pipe
(esophagus)

Esophageal
sphincter

Stomach

Stomach
contents

PART TWO

Causes, Symptoms, and Complications of GERD

In Part Two, we begin with a brief discussion of the anatomy and physiology of the gastrointestinal (GI) tract as it relates to GERD. We then discuss factors that influence transient LES relaxations, the principal cause of GERD. The main symptoms of GERD, heartburn and regurgitation are presented, as well as less common symptoms. Finally, the broad range of GERD complications is discussed.

CHAPTER 3
The Digestive Tract and GERD

CHAPTER 4
What Causes GERD?

CHAPTER 5
What Are the Symptoms of GERD?

CHAPTER 6
What are the Complications of GERD?

The Digestive Tract and GERD

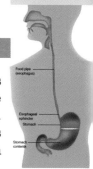

9. What actions in the mouth affect GERD?

Chewing food stimulates the release of saliva. Saliva serves as a lubricant to soften food, facilitating its passage through the digestive tract. It has a neutral pH (neither alkaline nor acidic). Saliva contains bicarbonate that can decrease the harmful effects of GERD by acting as a buffer, reducing a rise in acidity that can occur after the entry of acid refluxate into the esophagus.

10. What is the importance of the larynx and epiglottis?

Swallowing food is a complex process. After food is swallowed, it enters a passage known as the **pharynx**, where muscular contractions help move the bolus of food along until it reaches the **larynx**. The larynx is located at the juncture of the esophagus and trachea. The **trachea** or

To view a video on the gastrointestinal tract, visit:

https://www.youtube.com/watch?v=BHeSVxFONrQ

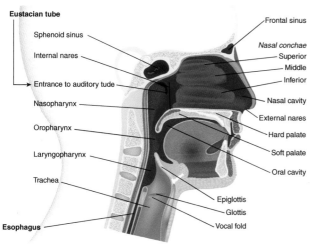

Eustacian tube
Sphenoid sinus
Internal nares
Entrance to auditory tude
Nasopharynx
Oropharynx
Laryngopharynx
Trachea
Esophagus

Frontal sinus
Nasal conchae
Superior
Middle
Inferior
Nasal cavity
External nares
Hard palate
Soft palate
Oral cavity
Epiglottis
Glottis
Vocal fold

The Upper Respiratory System

◀ **FIGURE 3.1**
The Upper Respiratory System

SOURCE: http://commons.wikimedia.org/wiki/File:Blausen_0872_UpperRespiratorySystem.png

AUTHOR: BruceBlaus-Creative Commons Attribution 3.0 Unported license windpipe is a tube that connects the throat to the lungs, allowing air to enter the lungs during breathing.

The larynx (also known as the voice box) consists of a cartilage skeleton housing the vocal cords. The larynx is covered by a flap of cartilage called the epiglottis. During breathing, the epiglottis is open, allowing air to pass into the trachea and lungs. When a person swallows, the epiglottis folds backward, covering the entrance of the trachea so that food and liquid do not enter the trachea and lungs. After passing the epiglottis, the food bolus enters the esophagus.

11. How does the esophagus function?

The esophagus is a muscular tube that serves as a conduit to transport food from the mouth into the stomach. The esophageal wall consists of four layers essential to its functioning (Kuo 2006).

The inner mucosal layer is an epithelium of squamous shaped cells that is exposed to the contents of the esophagus. This squamous epithelium is continuously sloughed off during the passage of food. The esophagus, contrary to the rest of the gastrointestinal tract, does not have a protective serosal coat over the mucosa. The absence of a serosal coat results in the esophagus being more vulnerable to the detrimental effects of acid reflux.

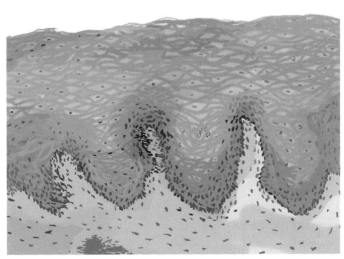

◄ FIGURE 3.2
Cross-section of normal epithelial lining showing flattened squamous shaped cells.

SOURCE: National Institute of Diabetes and Digestive and Kidney Diseases, National Institutes of Health.

The second layer is the **submucosa**, containing blood vessels, nerves, and glands.

The third layer, called the **muscularis**, consists of circular and longitudinal smooth muscle fibers. These muscles are involved in rhythmic peristaltic actions.

The fourth layer, called the **adventitia**, consists of fibrous connective tissue that covers the esophagus. Note that this layer is also called the serosa, but is distinct from serosa coating the epithelium in other parts of the digestive tract.

The passage of food through the esophagus stimulates nerves in the esophageal wall to induce rhythmic smooth muscle contractions that help to propel the food bolus through the esophagus. These contractions are known as peristalsis. As we shall see, peristalsis is also important to help return refluxate back into the stomach.

About 40–50% of GERD patients exhibit abnormal peristalsis, including low strength of peristalsis and slower propagation of peristaltic waves. It is unclear whether abnormal peristalsis is a condition that leads to GERD, or is a consequence of esophageal inflammation (Herbella 2010). Esophageal motility disorders, characterized by abnormal peristalsis, are discussed in Chapter 6.

▼ FIGURE 3.3
Layers of the Gastrointestinal Tract

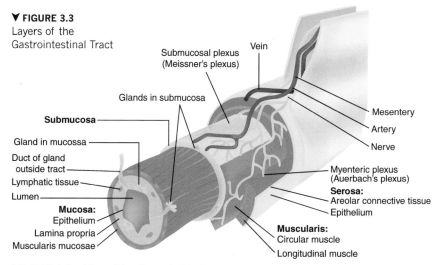

SOURCE: http://en.wikipedia.org/wiki/File:Layers_of_the_GI_Tract_english.svg

AUTHOR: Goran tek-en. Creative Commons Attribution-Share Alike 3.0 Unported license

The **esophagogastric sphincter** (EGS) is located at the point where the esophagus meets the stomach. The esophagogastric sphincter consists of the lower esophageal sphincter (LES) and the crural diaphragm.

The **lower esophageal sphincter** (LES) consists of two components (Mittal 1997). The circular and longitudinal muscle fibers of the esophagus extend into the sphincter. These smooth muscles are thicker in the sphincter, but the thickness is directly related to the sphincter pressure. The other component of the LES is the sling fibers of the fundus portion of the stomach. The sling fibers are curved in such a way (known as the **angle of His**) that pressure in the gastric fundus creates a flap that presses against the LES, thereby increasing the LES pressure and helping to prevent entry of stomach contents into the esophagus (Kapur 1998).

The diaphragm is a thin sheet of skeletal muscle that separates the thoracic cavity from the abdominal cavity. There are two types of diaphragmatic muscles: the **costal diaphragm** is involved in breathing, while the **crural diaphragm** also has a gastrointestinal function. The esophagus passes through an

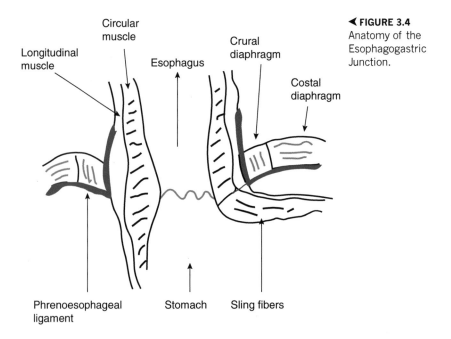

◄ **FIGURE 3.4**
Anatomy of the Esophagogastric Junction.

opening in the diaphragm known as the **hiatus** and the crural portion is attached to the lower esophageal sphincter by means of the phrenoesophageal ligament. The crural diaphragm is also known as the **external sphincter**.

The lower esophageal sphincter is the **internal sphincter**, and consists of a continuation of the smooth muscles of the esophagus (longitudinal and circular), and the sling fibers of the stomach. The crural diaphragm is the external sphincter. The two sphincters are joined by the phrenoesophageal ligament.

See companion files to watch a discussion of the pathophysiology of GERD and what treatments do or do not work.

https://www.youtube.com/watch?v=ojyFodct9kA

The LES (with assistance from the crural sphincter) serves as a valve that is normally closed as a result of tonic contraction of the sphincter muscles. As a result, positive pressure is maintained at the stomach side of the valve. When closed, reflux of stomach contents is prevented. The LES opens briefly and incompletely in response to swallowing and distension of the esophagus to permit passage of food boluses into the stomach. A reflex known as **transient LES relaxation** occurs to permit passage of gases generated in the stomach into the esophagus during belching. Transient LES relaxation can also result in the reflux of stomach contents into the esophagus.

13. How does the stomach function?

The stomach plays an important role in food digestion. The stomach lining is quite similar in structure and functioning to the esophageal lining. The mucosa, however, merits close examination. Instead of the squamous cells found in the esophagus, the stomach mucosa contains columnar epithelial cells which are more resistant to stomach acids. Within the epithelial lining are specialized cells that secrete digestive enzymes (pepsin and lipase), hydrochloric acid and mucus into the stomach lumen. The mixture of these secretions is known as gastric juice.

Digestion in the stomach takes place by a combination of chemical and mechanical digestion. Hydrochloric acid and pepsin act to digest proteins, lipase begins to digest fats, and mucus coats the lining of the stomach to protect it from gastric juice. Secretion of gastric juice begins as a nervous stimulation resulting

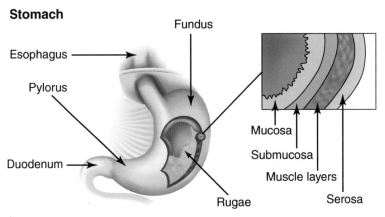

Stomach

Fundus

Esophagus

Pylorus

Duodenum

Rugae

Mucosa
Submucosa
Muscle layers
Serosa

▲ **FIGURE 3.5**
Illustration of parts of the stomach and the stomach lining. Note the esophagus passing through the hiatus opening in the diaphragm. The duodenum is the first part of the small intestine.

SOURCE: http://en.wikipedia.org/wiki/Gastrointestinal_wall "Illu stomach2," Licensed under Public Domain via Wikimedia Commons Creative Commons Public Domain Mark 1.0

For an animated look at the gastrointestinal tract, visit:

https://www.youtube.com/watch?v=BHeSVxFONrQ

ON THE WEB

from the process of eating, and continues as the bolus of food enters the stomach.

Peristaltic action is the mechanical phase which churns and mixes food with gastric juice to facilitate digestion.

14. Does digestion in the duodenum play a role in GERD?

The **duodenum** is the first part of the small intestine that is attached to the stomach through the **pyloric valve**. Digestive enzymes produced in the pancreas are secreted into the duodenum to bring about the digestion of proteins, fats, and carbohydrates. Additionally, bile is produced in the liver, and secreted via the bile duct into the duodenum. Bile aids in digestion of fats by physically breaking down fat into smaller particles called micelles.

Normally the pyloric valve is held tightly shut, preventing the entry of duodenal contents into the stomach. The valve opens briefly to allow stomach contents to enter the duodenum to continue digestion. Under some conditions (discussed later) the pyloric valve can open allowing duodenal contents to reflux into the stomach. This duodenal reflux will then mix with the stomach contents, becoming part of the non-acid reflux (Sifrim 2013).

What Causes GERD?

15. What causes GERD?

Several factors can lead to GERD and its complications (Levy 2002):

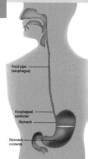

- Transient relaxations of the LES
- Consistently lower pressure of the LES
- Delayed emptying of gastric contents into the duodenum
- Delay in clearing of esophageal refluxate

Transient LES relaxations can occur when the stomach becomes distended after eating a large meal. Within the stomach wall are stretch receptors that are activated during stomach distension, causing transient LES relaxations (Holloway 1985, Penagini 2004). The stretching of the stomach has the effect of reducing the thickness of the stomach lining.

Consistently lower pressure of the LES can occur as a consequence of esophagitis or hiatal hernia. Often, the cause of consistently low pressure is unknown.

Eating fatty meals can be one reason for delayed emptying of gastric contents.

Faulty esophageal peristalsis can be an important reason for delayed movement of refluxate back into the stomach.

16. What is a hiatal hernia?

A **hiatal hernia** is a protrusion of part of the stomach through the hiatal opening. Hiatal hernia of the "sliding" type is by far the most common type, accounting for 95% of the cases. Sliding hiatal hernia is closely associated with GERD. Paraesophageal or "rolling" hiatal hernia accounts for 5% of the cases. Paraesophageal hiatal hernia may also be associated with GERD, but is more likely to cause serious complications. Hiatal hernia tends to increase with age, affecting about 60% of individuals in their 50s.

Several proposals have been brought forward to account for the appearance of hiatal hernias: 1) congenital defects of the esophagogastric junction, 2) traumatic injuries, and 3) increased abdominal pressures during pregnancy or straining to pass stool due to constipation (Sontag 1999).

Sliding hiatal hernia is thought to occur when there is a widening of the muscular hiatus and a weakening of the phrenoesophageal ligament. As a result, a part of the fundus portion of the stomach together with the LES slides through the hiatus into the thoracic cavity. The integrity of the esophagogastric junction is now destroyed as the LES is now separated from the crural membrane (Marks 2013). As a result, the two sphincters can no longer exert additive tonic contractions to prevent reflux. Additionally, the small pouch of stomach that is now above the diaphragm can trap acid coming from the stomach and keep it close to the esophagus. Finally, hiatal hernia can increase reflux by changing the angle of entry of the sling fibers. In hiatal hernia, this angle is straightened, resulting in the loss of the sling fiber's protective flap (Kahrilas 1999).

In paraesophageal hernias, a part of the gastric fundus also passes through the hiatal opening, remaining close to the esophagus, but the esophagogastric junction remains in place. In many people, paraesophageal hernias do not cause symptoms. If the hernia is large enough, it may press against the esophagus, hindering the free passage of food. Symptoms such as chest pain, upper abdominal pain, or difficulty swallowing indicate that the hernia may need to be repaired by surgery. Emergency surgery would be necessary if the stomach becomes obstructed by the hernia, or if its blood supply is cut off.

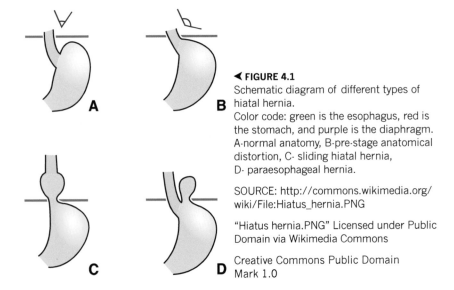

◄ **FIGURE 4.1**
Schematic diagram of different types of hiatal hernia.
Color code: green is the esophagus, red is the stomach, and purple is the diaphragm. A-normal anatomy, B-pre-stage anatomical distortion, C- sliding hiatal hernia, D- paraesophageal hernia.

SOURCE: http://commons.wikimedia.org/wiki/File:Hiatus_hernia.PNG

"Hiatus hernia.PNG" Licensed under Public Domain via Wikimedia Commons

Creative Commons Public Domain Mark 1.0

Peptic ulcers are breaks in the mucosal lining of the stomach (gastric ulcer) or the first part of the small intestine (duodenum). Peptic ulcers are the result of the burning action of acid and pepsin. There are many causes of peptic ulcers, including *H. pylori* infection, the use of NSAIDs, and conditions that cause increased secretion of acid.

Esophageal ulcers can be one of the complications of GERD, but they are not usually associated with peptic ulcers. Patients can confuse peptic ulcers with GERD, since the two conditions can exhibit similar symptoms. Treatment of the conditions can also be similar.

18. What is *H. pylori* infection, and can it cause GERD?

H. pylori is a bacterium that commonly infects the mucus lining of the stomach and small intestine. As the bacteria grow, they kill or damage the mucus producing cells resulting in a depletion of mucus lining. This loss of mucus lining allows acid and pepsin to reach the mucosal lining and cause ulcers. Although *H. pylori* is a major cause of peptic ulcers it does not really cause GERD; in fact, there is some evidence that *H. pylori* infection may actually decrease GERD (Peek 2004). If people are suffering from peptic ulcers, however, they should still definitely be tested for the presence of *H. pylori* regardless of their GERD status.

What are the Symptoms of GERD?

CHAPTER

5

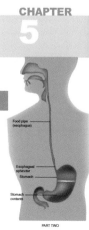

19. What is heartburn?

Heartburn, also known as **acid reflux**, is a characteristic symptom of GERD. It is often described as a burning pain in the middle of the chest, behind the breastbone, or in the upper part of the abdomen (Marks 2013). The pain occurs because nerve fibers in the esophagus are stimulated.

20. When is chest pain dangerous?

Many organs and tissues exist within the chest, all of which can be sources of pain. The heart, lungs, and esophagus are located in the chest behind the sternum or breastbone. The muscles of the rib cage could become sore and painful after vigorous exercise and hard physical work.

The name heartburn may have arisen from people who mistakenly confused the pain with a heart attack. *It is very important to have a physician diagnose any serious chest pain issue, because symptoms can vary among individuals and may not be typical.* The nerves supplying the heart also supply the esophagus, often making it difficult to distinguish the cause of chest pain based on symptoms.

Symptoms of a heart attack include a feeling of pressure, squeezing, fullness or pain in the center or left side of the chest. The feeling of pain or discomfort may spread to other parts of the body, and may be accompanied with shortness of breath. Other symptoms include irregular heart rate, dizziness, nausea, and unexplained sweating.

Acid reflux, on the other hand, can cause a burning sensation that remains localized. Patients with GERD can experience a temporary, intense chest pain when breathing deeply or coughing. Cardiac chest pain remains unchanged with deep breathing. GERD-related chest pain may be alleviated by changing your body position, while cardiac chest pain is not affected by body position. GERD-related chest pain can be intense when taking a deep breath or coughing. Symptoms are more common after meals, and can disturb sleep.

There are two other, less common causes of esophageal chest pain: spasms due to motility disorder and hypersensitivity of the esophagus. These conditions will be discussed in Chapter 6.

Several lung conditions can cause chest pain. Pleuritis or pleurisy is an inflammation or irritation of the lining surrounding the lungs and chest. Pleurisy causes a sharp pain when breathing, coughing, or sneezing. Pulmonary embolism is a blood clot that travels through the blood vessels and lodges in the lungs. The embolism can cause difficulty breathing in addition to severe pain. Pneumothorax occurs when a part of the lung collapses for any reason releasing air into the chest cavity. Pneumothorax can cause severe pain and difficulty breathing. The condition is life threatening.

CASE STUDY

Mark was a young man in his early 30s with a rising career as an executive in a major corporation. He decided to schedule a physical examination with his doctor because of episodes of burning and pain in the middle of his chest over the last six months. He was concerned about his health since he had a family history of heart disease. His father had a heart attack at 55 years of age, and both parents had long-term weight problems.

The doctor asked about Mark's lifestyle, and found out that he had a high-pressure job, ate poorly, and did not have an exercise program. The burning sensations usually occurred after meals, often accompanied by regurgitation. His voice occasionally became hoarse. He is overweight, but not obese. He took antacids occasionally as he thought his symptoms were due to indigestion. He experienced only a temporary improvement in his symptoms.

Although Mark's symptoms were strongly suggestive of GERD, his doctor ordered a complete cardiac examination, due to Mark's family history. Fortunately the cardiovascular workup indicated no heart disease. The cardiologist recommended changes in Mark's lifestyle to reduce his weight, including an improved diet and an exercise program.

Since Mark's symptoms did not indicate any GERD complication, Mark was given a prescription of omeprazole, a specific medication for GERD. The cardiologist's lifestyle recommendations were followed as they are beneficial for treating GERD as well.

After following the physicians' program for a month, Mark rarely had symptoms.

21. How can GERD cause regurgitation?

Regurgitation is the movement of refluxate from the esophagus up into the thorax and mouth. After eating large meals, there is a buildup of gases in the stomach. Regurgitation releases gases by burping or belching that involve transient LES relaxations. Regurgitation causes a sour taste in the mouth.

22. Why is regurgitation more dangerous while sleeping?

When you are awake, the swallowing reflex helps to move refluxate back down into the esophagus and stomach, and peristalsis is active to move refluxate from the esophagus back into the stomach. Swallowing brings down saliva and bicarbonate that protects the esophagus against refluxate. When you are sleeping, swallowing and peristalsis are inactive, so their protective effect is lost. Standing or sitting is more beneficial than lying down since gravity helps to keep gastric juice in the stomach.

23. What are other symptoms of GERD?

Other GERD symptoms include:

- a dry, chronic cough
- wheezing
- asthma and recurrent pneumonia
- nausea
- vomiting
- a sore throat, hoarseness, or laryngitis
- difficulty swallowing or painful swallowing
- pain in the chest or the upper part of the abdomen
- dental erosion and bad breath

These symptoms will be discussed in detail in Chapter 6.

24. What is dyspepsia and how is it related to GERD?

Dyspepsia is a term relating to symptoms originating from organs of the upper GI tract (esophagus, stomach, and duodenum). The common name for dyspepsia is indigestion, but the problem is probably not due to abnormal digestion of food. Symptoms of dyspepsia include pain or discomfort in the upper abdomen, bloating, belching, early satiety (sensation of fullness), and abdominal distension. Dyspepsia is commonly provoked by eating.

Theories of the causes of dyspepsia include an abnormal stimulation of the nerves and muscles that control the functioning of the esophagus, stomach, and duodenum (Marks 2014).

There are many causes of dyspepsia. The most common cases of dyspepsia are known as non-ulcer or functional dyspepsia, which occur in about 60% of affected people (Knott 2011). In functional dyspepsia, the upper GI tract appears normal by endoscopic examination.

Duodenal and stomach ulcers, as well as the inflammatory precursor conditions, duodenitis and gastritis, can be causes of dyspepsia.

GERD and hiatus hernia can be causes, as may be apparent from some of the indicated symptoms.

Anti-inflammatory medicines and various other medicines can also be culprits.

Finally, stomach and esophageal cancer can cause dyspepsia when they first develop.

We present this discussion of dyspepsia due to its close association to GERD. In fact, many of the diagnostic tools and treatments for dyspepsia are similar to those for GERD.

25. Can GERD occur without any symptoms?

Each person can react differently to acid reflux, and may not experience heartburn. Refluxate can also regurgitate unnoticed into the pharynx, mouth, and trachea where it can cause problems as discussed in Chapter 6.

What are the Complications of GERD?

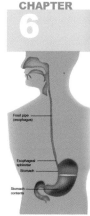

CHAPTER

6

Esophageal complications of GERD include esophagitis, stricture, esophageal motility disorder, esophageal hypersensitivity, Barrett's esophagus and adenocarcinoma. Extraesophageal complications (above the esophagus) include chronic cough, laryngitis, asthma, dental lesions, and ear and nose symptoms. These complications can occur in up to 50% of patients exhibiting acid reflux (Yuksel 2012).

26. What is esophagitis?

Esophagitis is a general term for any inflammation, irritation, or swelling of the esophagus. Esophagitis can range from mild redness, to erosion, and to ulceration of the mucosa.

27. What is esophageal stricture?

Esophageal stricture (also called peptic stricture) is a narrowing of the esophageal lumen (the inner open space) often resulting in dysphagia (difficulty in swallowing). It has been estimated that 70–80% of all cases of esophageal stricture are due to GERD. Peptic stricture is considered to be the end stage of reflux disease (Mukherjee 2012). Chronic acid reflux leads to inflammation, fibrosis (scarring), and narrowing of the lining and wall of the esophagus. Esophagitis is an important cause of dysphasia independent of the degree of stricture. A large percentage of patients with strictures also have hiatal hernias. Strictures are usually benign, but will progress in time if GERD is untreated. Esophagitis and stricture is more common in older patients.

If dysphagia becomes a serious problem, esophageal stricture can be treated by dilation at the time of an endoscopy procedure. (Endoscopy will be discussed in Chapter 10.) The overall frequency of dilation procedures have decreased after the introduction of GERD medications known as proton pump inhibitors. Physicians have had considerable success in treating and managing dysphasia by lifestyle and dietary changes in addition to medications without resorting to surgery.

28. What are esophageal motility disorders?

As discussed, esophageal peristalsis is a fine-tuned affair, requiring the close coordination of nerves and muscles to rapidly and efficiently propel the food bolus from the pharynx to the stomach. Esophageal motility disorders encompass a broad class of diseases that are manifested by abnormal contractions of the esophagus as well as by abnormal functioning of both the upper and lower esophageal sphincters (Diener 2001). Motility is a biological term simply meaning movement.

Esophageal spasms are an outcome of the disorder and consist of two main types:

- Diffuse esophageal spasm is irregular, uncoordinated peristalsis that prevents food from reaching the stomach. Food is stuck in the esophagus leading to dysphasia.
- Nutcracker esophagus is coordinated but very strong peristaltic contractions that can cause severe chest pain.

Other disorders include ineffective esophageal motility resulting in decreased strength of peristaltic contractions, and achalasia, which results in complete loss of peristalsis. Both conditions lead to dysphasia.

The causes of esophageal motility disorders are largely not known. The inflammation and scarring resulting from acid reflux that damage the nerves and muscles of the esophageal wall could be one cause.

Esophageal motility disorders can be diagnosed by manometry (discussed in Chapter 10).

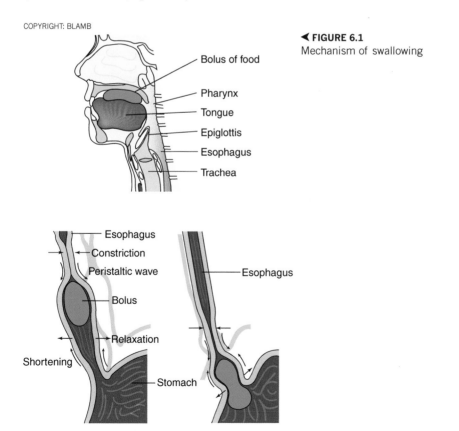

◄ FIGURE 6.1
Mechanism of swallowing

Bolus of food

Pharynx

Tongue

Epiglottis

Esophagus

Trachea

Esophagus

Constriction

Peristaltic wave

Esophagus

Bolus

Relaxation

Shortening

Stomach

People with esophageal hypersensitivity (Gyawali 2010) have an abnormal sensory or pain response to stimuli such as distension or contraction of the esophagus or to acid or other chemical agents. The condition is also known as an irritable esophagus. Hypersensitivity can manifest as either a painful response to normally non-painful stimuli, or an increased pain response to stimuli that are normally painful. Esophageal hypersensitivity may be associated with esophageal motility disorder.

Hypersensitivity is a dysregulation of the pathway leading from the esophageal lining where the receptors are located, through connections between the esophagus and the brain, to the brain's perception of the sensory information.

The causes for esophageal hypersensitivity are uncertain, but can include triggers such as acid reflux and other noxious chemicals damaging the epithelium. In addition, psychological issues including anxiety, depression and panic disorders may contribute to heightened pain sensitivity. The relationship of stress to GERD is discussed in Question 44.

Esophageal rings are thin, narrow extensions of mucosal and submucosal tissue that encircle the esophageal lumen, usually a few centimeters above the esophagogastric junction. The most common rings are called Schatzki rings, and are almost always associated with hiatal hernia. Esophageal webs are thin membranes that extend into the lumen, and are of similar origin. Controversy exists whether esophageal rings and webs are hereditary, or whether they form as a consequence of acid reflux.

Most patients with rings and webs do not have symptoms, but when the lumen opening decreases to 13–20 millimeters, dysphasia is likely to occur. Patients with mild dysphasia are advised to modify their eating habits by eating soft food, cutting food into small pieces, and eating slowly. The term steakhouse syndrome is based on the story of a restaurant patron rapidly swallowing a large portion of steak, only to have the piece lodged in his esophagus at the point where the ring occurs. The person

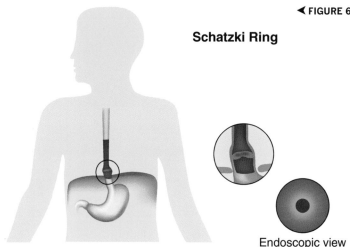

Schatzki Ring

Endoscopic view

SOURCE: Alila Medical Media/Shutterstock.com

may have to vomit up the food in order to clear the blockage, or may even need to visit the emergency room.

Similar to esophageal strictures, rings can be treated during an endoscopy procedure.

31. What is Barrett's esophagus?

Esophagitis usually heals by regeneration of normal epithelial squamous cells. In some individuals, however, the squamous cells are replaced by columnar shaped cells typical of the small intestine. This process, known as **Barrett's esophagus**, results in epithelial cells that are more resistant to the effects of reflux acids. Barrett's esophagus is characterized by abnormal "tongues" of salmon colored mucosa extending from the gastro-esophageal junction into the normal pale esophageal mucosa (Enzinger 2003).

There are no characteristic symptoms of Barrett's esophagus apart from GERD. The condition is a result of chronic esophagitis, and is discovered during endoscopy, a procedure undertaken to diagnose GERD symptoms.

Barrett's esophagus develops in approximately 5–8% of patients with GERD. Barrett's esophagus involves a process known as metaplasia making the

DEFINITION

Metaplasia is a change in the type of adult cells in a tissue to another form of adult cells that are not normal for that tissue.

individual 40-fold more susceptible to adenocarcinoma compared with the general population.

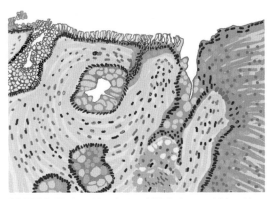

◀ **FIGURE 6.3**
Cross section of esophageal lining showing development of columnar shaped epithelial cells in Barrett's esophagus.

SOURCE: National Institute of Diabetes and Digestive and Kidney Diseases, National Institutes of Health.

32. How do you monitor and treat Barrett's esophagus in patients?

A diagnosis of Barrett's esophagus is a serious matter, given the risk of its progression to esophageal cancer. This situation requires that a patient with Barrett's must be monitored on a regular basis.

The epithelial cells of Barrett's can be graded according to their degree of abnormality, or **dysplasia**. Non-dysplastic Barrett's esophagus cells have no abnormalities in size, shape, or organization. Low-grade dysplasia and high-grade dysplasia indicate progressively greater abnormalities.

Professional gastroenterology associations have established guidelines for monitoring Barrett's esophagus by means of endoscopy and biopsy. Patients diagnosed with non-dysplastic Barrett's should have another endoscopy a year later to ensure no changes have taken place. If higher grades of dysplasia are found, endoscopies are taken more frequently.

If Barrett's esophagus progresses to a high-grade dysplasia, therapies should be considered. Without treatment, invasive cancer reportedly develops within three years in up to half of patients with high-grade dysplasia. Previously, the only effective therapy was removal of the esophagus. However, this procedure is very traumatic with a morbidity rate of 40–50%. Recently, radiofrequency ablation has become a well-accepted procedure that is routinely performed (Massachusetts General Hospital 2014). Ablation has the beneficial outcome of reversing the abnormal columnar epithelial cells of Barrett's esophagus back to normal squamous cells. The procedure is discussed in Question 86.

33. What is adenocarcinoma?

There are two main types of esophageal cancer: squamous cell carcinoma and adenocarcinoma. **Squamous cell carcinoma** is found in the upper part of the esophagus (near the larynx) and may be related to heavy alcohol consumption or smoking. **Adenocarcinoma** is found in the lower part of the esophagus, and is associated with GERD.

Common symptoms of patients with esophageal cancer include dysphagia, pain on swallowing food and liquids, and weight loss. Dyspenia (shortness of breath), cough, hoarseness, and pain may be present in patients with advanced esophageal cancer.

Patients with recurring symptoms of acid reflux have a nearly eightfold increased risk of adenocarcinoma (Lagergren et al. 1999), while the risk of any given patient developing adenocarcinoma in a year is approximately one in 200. The lifetime risk of all types of esophageal cancer is low, however: 0.8% for men and 0.3% for women. Studies have suggested that the incidence of adenocarcinoma has increased 300–500% throughout the last 30–40 years (Nicolas 2002).

The initial diagnosis of adenocarcinoma is often obtained by an **esophagogram**, which can show a stricture or ulceration of the esophagus. A follow-up upper endoscopy study can reveal a friable, ulcerated mass. Other studies are performed to determine the stage of the cancer and whether it has spread (metastasized).

If esophageal cancer is detected at an early stage, the tumor can be removed surgically with an excellent prognosis. If the cancer has spread, chemotherapy and radiation therapies are performed. Unfortunately, more than 50% of patients have an advanced stage of cancer at the time of detection resulting in a grim prognosis. The overall five-year survival rate for esophageal cancer is low, around 17% (Enzinger 2003).

For the following upper respiratory tract complications, please refer back to Figure 3.1- the Upper Respiratory Tract.

NOTE

Aspiration is the drawing up of microdroplets of refluxate into the larynx and trachea. As mentioned, refluxate enters the upper esophagus and pharynx by the process of regurgitation. Aspiration is more likely to occur at night as the act of breathing opens the epiglottis allowing refluxate droplets to enter the trachea together with air.

Aspiration is very serious as the refluxate droplets irritate the larynx and trachea potentially leading to chronic cough, laryngitis, and aspiration pneumonia, as well as aggravating the symptoms of allergy. Controversy exists within the scientific community as to whether the aggravating factor is acid or pepsin (Bardhan 2012, Johnson 2013).

35. How can GERD cause chronic cough and laryngitis?

Chronic cough is a cough of more than eight weeks duration.

DEFINITION

Regurgitation can result in aspiration of microdroplets of refluxate into the larynx and pharynx, causing cough as a protective mechanism against reflux. In this case, the more correct term is **laryngopharyngeal reflux** (LPR). Reports indicate that 25% or more of chronic cough cases are associated with GERD, although this does not necessarily mean that GERD is the cause of the chronic cough in many of these individuals (Madanick 2013).

Chronic cough may occur in individuals without the usual GERD symptoms of heartburn and regurgitation. This group of patients tends not to respond well to acid suppressive therapy. The finding that weakly acidic reflux can cause chronic cough has led some physicians to believe that pepsin is the culprit.

Laryngitis is an inflammation of the larynx or voice box. Laryngitis includes the symptoms of hoarseness, throat pain, sensation of a lump in the throat, cough, repetitive throat clearing, excessive phlegm, difficulty swallowing, pain with swallowing, and loss of voice. Acute laryngitis is due to infection, while chronic (long lasting) laryngitis is due to LPR, post-nasal drip, allergens, smoking, and other environmental pollutants.

36. What is relationship of GERD to asthma?

Asthma is a chronic disease that inflames and narrows the airways, which serve as conduits to transport gases to and from the lungs. Asthma is a very common disease affecting more than 25 million people in the U.S. (National Heart Association 2014). The exact cause of asthma is not known. Researchers think some genetic and environmental factors interact to cause asthma. Most people with asthma also develop allergies.

An asthma attack is caused by triggering factors that irritate the airways resulting in tightening and swelling of the airways, with the formation of thick mucus. All of these triggering factors result in a narrowing of the airways causing difficulty in breathing. The triggering factors can include respiratory infections, allergens, irritants, and some medicines.

GERD can provoke asthma attacks when refluxate is aspirated into the airways and irritates the trachea. Asthma in turn can cause reflux due to a reduction of pressure within the chest cavity (Yuksel E 2012).

37. Can GERD cause injury to the teeth?

When regurgitation of acid reflux reaches the mouth, it can cause a sour taste. It is well established that the highly acidic nature of the refluxate can dissolve the enamel of the teeth resulting in erosion (Pace 2008). The reduced salivary secretion occurring with GERD results in a lowered protective buffering effect against acid. The prevalence of GERD in patients with dental erosion can range from 21 to 83%. It should be noted that GERD has no detrimental effect on the development of dental caries.

38. Can GERD affect the nose, sinuses, and inner ear?

The upper portion of the pharynx, known as the nasopharynx, has direct connections to the nose, sinuses, and ears. The inner ears are connected to the nasopharynx by means of the Eustachian tubes. The function of the Eustachian tubes is to equalize atmospheric and inner ear pressures. Inflammation and fluid accumulation in the tubes as a result of exposure to refluxate could partially block the tubes, compromising its functioning and leading to inner ear discomfort. Since Eustachian tube dysfunction is more frequent in children, ear manifestations due to GERD are nearly exclusive to children (Caruso 2006).

Nose and sinus manifestations as a result of acid reflux are also more frequent in children. The mechanism by which GERD affects the nose and sinuses is unclear, but is likely due to inflammation, fluid accumulation, and blockage of the nasal and sinus cavities.

Sinuses are hollow cavities located in the bones of the skull and face. Sinuses are connected to the nasal passages by small tubes or channels. Sinuses and their passages are coated with mucus membranes.

It is important to note that GERD is only one of many possible causes of problems to the nose, sinuses, and inner ears.

39. What is non-acid reflux and how is it related to GERD complications?

The refluxate entering the esophagus contains of all the stomach contents. Although acid is perceived to be the most detrimental component of the refluxate, non-acid components such as pepsin and bile can also be detrimental (Tack 2006). We have discussed how pepsin, derived from stomach secretions, could either increase the detrimental effect of acid, or could be independently detrimental. Bile, which is involved in duodenal digestion, can also be detrimental.

Normally, the pyloric valve remains strongly closed to prevent reflux of duodenal contents into the stomach. This reflux is commonly called bile reflux, but it also contains other components such as pancreatic enzymes.

Conditions that injure the pyloric valve and prevent its proper functioning could permit the entry of bile reflux into the stomach. Once in the stomach, the bile reflux will mix with stomach contents. Conditions that could compromise pyloric valve functioning include severe GERD, peptic ulcer, and stomach surgery.

Why should you be concerned about bile reflux? The most popular GERD medications focus on acid reduction. If these medications fail to alleviate symptoms, it could indicate that non-acid reflux still passing through the LES is continuing to cause injury.

We have discussed how acid reflux damages the esophagus, leading to inflammation. A recent study (Reveiller 2012) found that bile is also likely to be a cause of esophageal inflammation. The study found that bile is responsible for the changes in epithelial lining characteristic of Barrett's esophagus. As mentioned, epithelial lining is continuously sloughed off and replaced by new tissue. Bile apparently has the ability to shut off genes responsible for growing squamous cells, and turning on genes that grow columnar cells. Recall that columnar epithelial cells are normal for the duodenum (the environment in which bile normally operates).

How can bile reflux be treated? The best treatment method is to block all reflux components from entering the esophagus by strengthening LES functioning. One possibility is the use of baclofen (described in Question 78), which reduces transient LES relaxations. Also in Chapter 11, we will discuss how some antacid formulations contain alginates. Alginates can bind to the esophageal mucosa, inhibiting the diffusion and activity of pepsin. However, the use of alginates (other than those present in antacid medications) have not received much attention. Surgery to correct the LES is the final recourse.

References

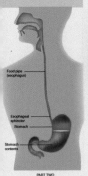

CHAPTER 3

1   Herbella, Fernando A., and Marco G. Patti. "Gastroesophageal reflux disease: From pathophysiology to treatment." *World Journal of Gastroenterology* 16, no. 30 (August 14, 2010): 3745–3749.

2   Kapur Kapil C., Nigel J. Trudgill, and Stuart A. Riley. "Mechanisms of gastro-oesophageal reflux in the lateral decubitus positions." *Neurogastroenterology & Motility* 10, no. 6 (December 1998): 517–522.

3   Kuo, Braden, and Daniela Urma. (2006). "Esophagus-anatomy and development." *GI Motility Online* (2006). Retrieved May 16, 2006, from http://www.nature.com/gimo/contents/pt1/full/gimo6.html.

4   Mittal, Ravinder K., Hubert A. Shaffer, Stella Parollisi, and Lane Baggett. "Influence of breathing pattern on the esophagogastric junction pressure and esophageal transit." *American Journal of Physiology* 269, no. 4 Part 1 (1995): G577–G583.

5   Sifrim, Daniel. "Management of Bile Reflux." *Gastroenterology & Hepatology* 9 no. 3 (March 2013): 179–180.

CHAPTER 4

6   Holloway, Richard H., Michio Hongo, Keith Berger, and Richard W. McCallum. "Gastric distention: a mechanism for postprandial gastroesophageal reflux." *Gastroenterology* 89, no. 4 (October 1985): 779–84.

7   Kahrilas, Peter. (1999). "The Role of Hiatus Hernia in GERD." *Yale Journal of Biology and Medicine* 72, nos. 2–3 (1999): 101–11.

8   Levy, Robyn A., Linda Stamm, and Sue E. Meiner. "Conservative Management of GERD: A Case Study." *MEDSURG Nursing* 11, no. 4 (2002): 169–75.

9   Marks, Jay W., and Charles Patrick Davis. "Gastroesophageal Reflux Disease." MedicineNet.com (2013), http://www.medicinenet.com/gastroesophageal_reflux_disease_gerd/article.htm.

10   Peek, Richard M. "Helicobacter pylori and Gastroesophageal Reflux Disease." *Current Treatment Options in Gastroenterology* 7, no. 1 (2004): 59–70.

11   Penagini, Roberto, Stefania Carmagnola, Paolo Cantù, Mariangela Allocca, and Paolo A. Bianchi. "Mechanoreceptors of the proximal stomach: Role in triggering transient lower esophageal sphincter relaxation." *Gastroenterology* 126, no. 1(January 2004): 49–56.

12   Sontag, Stephen J. "Defining GERD." *Yale Journal of Biology and Medicine* 72, nos. 2–3 (1999): 69–80.

CHAPTER 5

13 Knott, Laurence. "Dyspepsia (Indigestion)." Patient.co.uk. Document ID: 4868 (v42), 2011. http://www.patient.co.uk/health/ dyspepsia-indigestion

15 Marks Jay W., and Charles Patrick Davis. "Indigestion (Dyspepsia), Upset Stomach." MedicineNet.com, 2014. http://www.medicinenet .com/dyspepsia/article.htm

CHAPTER 6

17 Bardhan, Karna Dev, Vicki Strugala, and Peter W. Dettmar (2012). "Reflux Revisited: Advancing the Role of Pepsin." International Journal of Otolaryngology (2012), Article ID 646901. http:// www.ncbi.nlm.nih.gov/pmc/articles/PMC3216344/pdf/ IJOL2012-646901.pdf

18 Caruso Giuseppe, and Francesco Maria Passàli. (2006). "ENT manifestations of gastro-oesophageal reflux in children." Acta Otorhinolaryngologica Italica 26 (2006): 252–5.

19 Diener, Urs, Marco G. Patti, Daniela Molena, Piero M. Fisichella, and Lawrence W. Way. "Esophageal dysmotility and gastroesophageal reflux disease." *Journal of Gastrointestinal Surgery* 5, no. 3 (2001): 260–5.

20 Enzinger, Peter, and Robert Mayer. "Esophageal Cancer." *New England Journal of Medicine* 349, no 23 (2003): 2241–52.

21 Gyawali, Chandra. "Esophageal Hypersensitivity." *Gastroenterology & Hepatology* 6, no. 8 (August 2010): 497–500.

22 Johnson, David A. "The Dreaded Diagnosis of Laryngopharyngeal Reflux Disease." Medscape, January 29, 2013. http://www .medscape.com/viewarticle/778052

23 Lagergren, Jesper, Reinhold Bergström, Anders Lindgren, and Olof Nyrén. "Symptomatic gastroesophageal reflux as a risk factor for esophageal adenocarcinoma." *New England Journal of Medicine* 340 (1999): 825–31.

24 Madanick, Ryan. "Management of GERD-Related Chronic Cough." *Gastroenterology & Hepatology* 9, no. 5 (May 2013): 311–3.

25 Massachusetts General Hospital. "Radiofrequency Ablation Treatment for Barrett's Esophagus" (2014). http://www .massgeneral.org/digestive/services/procedure.aspx?id=2298

26 Mukherjee, Sandeep. "Esophageal Stricture." *Medscape*, Updated January 4, 2012. http://emedicine.medscape.com/article/ 175098-overview

27 Pace, Fabio, Stefano Pallotta, Marcello Tonini, Nimish Vakil, and Gabriele Bianchi Porro. "Systematic review: Gastro-oesophageal reflux disease and dental lesions." *Alimentary Pharmacology & Therapeutics* 27 (2008): 1179–86.

28 Reveiller, Marie, Sayak Ghatak, Liana Toia, Irina Kalatskaya, Lincoln Stein, Mary D'Souza, Zhongren Zhou, Santhoshi Bandla, William E Gooding, Tony E Godfrey, Jeffrey H Peters. "Bile Exposure Inhibits Expression of Squamous and Differentiation Genes in Human Esophageal Epithelial Cells." *Annals of Surgery* 255, no. 6 (June 2012):1113–20.

29 Shaheen, Nicholas J., and David J. Frantz. "When to Consider Endoscopic Ablation Therapy for Barrett's Esophagus." *Current Opinion in Gastroenterology* 26, no .4 (2010): 361–6.

30 Tack, Jan. "Review article: the role of bile and pepsin in the pathophysiology and treatment of gastro-oesophageal reflux disease." *Alimentary Pharmacology & Therapeutics* 24, Suppl. 2 (2006): 10–16.

31 Yuksel, Elif Saritas, and Michael Vaezi. "Extraesophageal manifestations of gastroesophageal reflux disease: cough, asthma, laryngitis, chest pain." *Swiss Medical Weekly* 142 (2012): w13544.

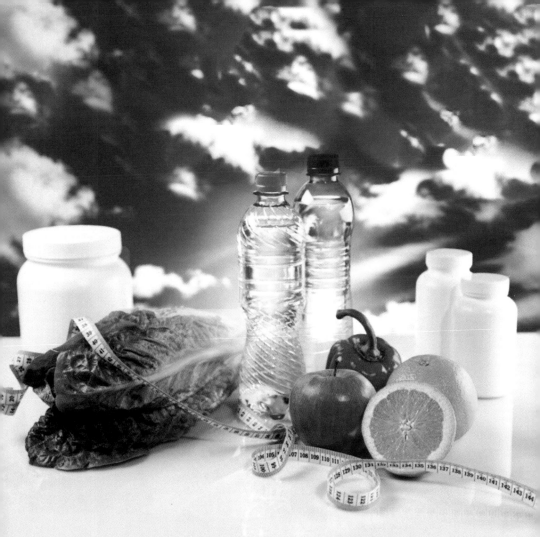

PART THREE

The influence of lifestyle modifications, certain foods, and medications on the occurrence of GERD

In Part Three, we discuss lifestyle modifications, the first steps usually taken to reduce the severity of GERD. We discuss how certain lifestyle modifications such as exercise, cessation of smoking, reduction of body weight, and avoiding certain foods can help in reducing GERD symptoms. We then discuss how certain medications used for purposes other than GERD may adversely affect GERD.

CHAPTER 7
How does a person's lifestyle affect GERD?

CHAPTER 8
What foods and beverages make GERD worse?

CHAPTER 9
What drugs and medications make GERD worse?

How does a person's lifestyle affect GERD?

40. What are the most common factors that trigger GERD symptoms?

Participants in a survey indicated that meals were by far the most common trigger for GERD symptoms (80%), followed by stress (around 30%), and physical activity (around 15%) (Jones 2007).

41. Does obesity affect GERD?

Obesity has been characterized as reaching "epidemic proportions" in Western societies. Obesity is linked to the development of GERD and complications such as adenocarcinoma (esophageal cancer). The associations are stronger in women than men, and stronger in white populations than in other ethnic populations (Lagergren 2011).

Several physiological mechanisms have been proposed to account for the relationship of obesity to GERD. Obesity can be measured by such means as body mass index (BMI) and waist circumference. Many studies have shown positive associations between these measures of obesity and GERD (Festi 2009). It has been proposed that increased waist circumference leads to increased pressure within the abdomen and stomach. Increased stomach distension leads to more transient LES relaxations. Additionally, obesity is associated with a separation of the LES from the crural diaphragm, predisposing obese patients to hiatal hernia. Obesity, as measured by BMI, shows a stronger association with GERD among premenopausal women compared with postmenopausal women, suggesting an influence of estrogen exposure. Studies have shown a direct relationship between obesity and esophagitis (Festi 2009).

Will weight reduction alleviate GERD in obese patients?

Based on many studies, weight loss by diet or surgery appears to hold promise, but the results are not consistent.

Some severely obese persons resort to bariatric surgery, which involves reducing the size of the stomach in order to reduce intake of food and absorption of nutrients. These procedures may have a side benefit of reducing GERD, but the surgery is too traumatic to be undertaken specifically for that purpose.

Regardless of its effect on GERD, weight reduction has very important benefits for people who are overweight or obese. Weight reduction is a vast subject, but it suffices to say that a combination of correct diet, exercise, and stress reduction can be beneficial to general health as well as for reducing GERD.

42. Can smoking aggravate symptoms of GERD?

Smokers have higher rates of reflux symptoms than nonsmokers, according to the results of questionnaires and analyses of case-control studies (Kaltenbach 2006). There is a direct association between the duration of tobacco smoking and the risk of reflux symptoms. Although smoking appears to decrease LES pressure, smokers may not show increased esophageal acid exposure time.

Smoking has several detrimental effects that can increase the severity of GERD. Cigarette smoke can dry out the mouth, resulting in decreased salivary bicarbonate secretion. The reduced presence of bicarbonate in the esophagus could result in reduced neutralizing of esophageal acid (Meining 2000). Smoking can increase transient LES relaxations (Talalwah 2013). Cigarette smoke can augment irritation of the esophagus in the presence of acid reflux. Finally, smoking greatly increases the risk of esophageal cancer.

The case-control study described here compares cases of individuals with GERD to control individuals without the disease and looks for differences in prior exposure to smoking either through medical records or patient recall.

Will smoking cessation reduce symptoms? A literature review indicated only limited effectiveness.

43. How does exercise affect GERD?

Exercise has general health benefits, and the usual recommendation is for a person to participate in at least 30 minutes of exercise for most days of the week. However, the intensity, duration, and type of exercises can affect GERD and may make it worse. Vigorous exercise, such as running, cycling, and weight lifting may induce reflux symptoms (Festi 2009). Exercises that involve abdominal straining can put pressure on the stomach, and may distort the esophagogastric junction.

A person with GERD should not forego the benefits of exercise, but should take a few necessary precautions. The person should not exercise after meals to allow time for digestion to take place. The stomach should be empty or nearly empty prior to exercise. Fatty foods that are slow to digest should be avoided prior to exercising. Sports or carbonated drinks should be avoided, and the person should only drink water while exercising. Through experience, the individual will learn about the exercises that will trigger GERD and that should be avoided. The key point is moderation in exercise.

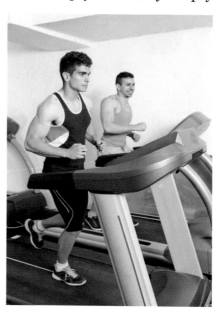

Long-term exercise programs could reduce GERD if they result in weight reduction in obese patients.

44. Does stress increase GERD symptoms?

The stress response developed in early man as a means of coping with physical threats to his existence. When the senses perceive a danger, various neurological and hormonal responses take place in the body to prepare the person to cope with the danger. Although physical threats still exist for modern man, quite often stress is psychologically based. When this happens, the stress response no longer serves its original purpose to gear up the person to confront the stress by "fight or flight." In this situation, stress can become chronic, with detrimental effects on the body.

Stress may exacerbate GERD by several mechanisms. One of the characteristics of the stress response is the shutdown of the digestive process. This effect can result in the slowing of gastric emptying leading to an accumulation of gastric acid. As we will discuss, decreasing stomach acid is a primary goal of GERD treatment. Stress may increase transient LES relaxations. Stress may alter a person's breathing pattern, causing increased tension on the crural diaphragm, and changed functioning of the esophagogastric junction. One result could be incomplete esophageal clearance of acid refluxate (Mittal 1995).

Stress can also be related to GERD in indirect ways. Stress can cause weight gain due to an increased craving for comfort foods high in salt, fat, and sugar. These cravings may be due to an increased secretion of the hormone cortisol during stress (New York Times 2013).

> A certain amount of stress in life is normal and inevitable. If you are concerned your stress is affecting your health or is aggravating your GERD, a vast amount of literature is available that discuss ways to reduce stress. A good place to start is on the NIH Health Information website:
>
> http://health.nih.gov/search_results.aspx

ON THE WEB

It has been apparent that people experiencing stress and other psychological symptoms report a worsening of GERD symptoms. This is known as **comorbidity** (Mizyed 2009). The worsening of symptoms may be due to esophageal hypersensitivity (discussed previously), which is a further complication of acid reflux (Mayer 2000).

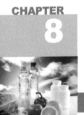

CHAPTER 8 *What foods and beverages make GERD worse?*

45. What is a "GERD diet?"

The effect of certain foods, food ingredients, and beverages on GERD is very much a personal matter. One person can experience severe reflux to a certain food, while the food can have no effect on another person. This variability is probably the reason that research studies rarely show significant effects of certain foods on GERD symptoms.

Of course, this is no reason for you to dismiss the effect of diet on GERD. Your doctor will probably make dietary recommendations, knowing that dietary changes may affect GERD, and may make the medicines he or she prescribes more effective.

An excellent way to develop your personalized "GERD diet" is to maintain a food diary for several weeks, writing down what you eat, when you eat it, and any symptoms you may experience. You may find out that your symptoms may vary depending on your emotional state, eating too fast or overeating, or eating just before bedtime.

46. What beverages affect reflux?

Alcoholic beverages can increase GERD through several mechanisms. Alcohol increases acid secretion in the stomach by stimulating release of the hormone gastrin, by increasing transient LES relaxations, by reducing LES pressure, and by impairing esophageal movements, and by emptying the stomach. Some studies show no association, however (Nilsson 2003).

Alcohol may increase GERD symptoms due to a direct toxic effect on the esophageal mucosa (Meining 2000). Studies have indicated that alcohol users have a greater prevalence of GERD symptoms. A review of the literature, however, indicated that there is no evidence that reducing alcohol consumption will decrease reflux symptoms (Talalwah 2013).

Carbonated beverages can release gas in the stomach. This excess gas may increase GERD symptoms through belching by causing transient LES relaxations. The current literature, however, has not shown evidence that carbonated beverages promote or exacerbate GERD (Johnson 2010). Carbonated beverages may indirectly contribute to GERD by promoting obesity.

Citrus juices can provoke reflux in some people, but the citrus effect on GERD may be due to factors in addition to acidity (Meining 2000, Kaltenbach 2006).

Large studies have shown conflicting evidence on the role of coffee drinking on GERD. Many large studies have found no association between coffee or tea consumption and GERD (Festi 2009).

47. Can certain foods aggravate GERD?

Foods that may aggravate GERD include:

a. Fatty and fried foods are slower to digest and remain in the stomach longer. When stomach emptying is delayed, acid can accumulate in the gastric juice. Examples include:

- fatty cuts of meat and bacon
- fatty dairy products, such as cheese, cream, and butter
- French fries and onion rings
- high-fat desserts such as ice cream and potato chips
- cream sauces, gravies, and creamy salad dressings
- chicken nuggets, buffalo wings

b. Tomatoes and citrus fruits are acidic foods and may increase acid in the stomach. Examples include:

- tomatoes and tomato sauce
- salsa
- chili
- pizza
- oranges
- grapefruit
- limes
- lemons
- pineapple

c. Garlic and onions

d. Condiments

- strong mustard
- chili sauces
- creamy salad dressing
- black pepper
- pickles
- curries

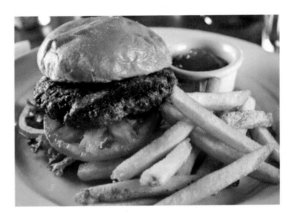

▶ FIGURE 8.1
Fatty and fried foods can increase GERD in some people

Many foods can be chosen for your GERD diets that do not aggravate GERD (Griffin 2013):

a. Fruits that are low in acidity include:

- apples
- bananas
- pears
- peaches
- melons
- strawberries
- melons

b. Green and root vegetables

- baked potato
- broccoli
- carrots
- green beans
- peas
- asparagus
- lettuce
- sweet potatoes

c. Lean meats can be good choices (prepare grilled, broiled, baked, or steamed—not fried)

- lean ground beef and steaks
- chicken breast
- turkey meat
- fish

d. Low-fat dairy products

- skim or 1% milk
- fat-free cream cheese or sour cream
- feta or goat cheese

e. Grains

- bran cereals
- oatmeal

- brown rice
- quinoa
- whole grain bread
- hummus

f. Condiments

- low-fat salad dressing .
- fennel
- parsley
- ginger
- aloe vera

49. Is meal size and timing of meals important?

It is a common belief that large meals can cause acid reflux. Strengthening this belief is the observation that stomach distension triggers transient LES relaxations. Although there have not yet been adequate studies to investigate the effect of large meals on reflux, it is still recommended that large meals be avoided (Meining 2000).

GERD symptoms are most often provoked after eating, indicating a close relationship between foods and GERD. An important principle to follow is to eat slowly, and not overeat. In this manner, digestion can proceed efficiently and completely.

50. How should GERD patients manage bedtime?

It is generally recommended that meals should not be eaten within about three hours before going to bed, and that GERD patients keep the head in an elevated position while in bed. Raising the head of the bed is apparently more effective than the use of extra pillows. This advice is due to observation that the stomach and esophagus are at the same level while lying down making it more difficult for acid and stomach contents to leave the esophagus. The American College of Gastroenterology supports these recommendations.

Evidence has shown that lying on the left side results in less acid reflux than lying on the right side. Although the reasons are unclear, reflux may occur more frequently on the right because the stomach contents lie in closer proximity to the gastroesophageal junction (Kapur 1998).

CASE STUDY

George, a white male in his late 40s, visited his doctor with complaints of acid reflux. For the past month, he has had a burning sensation with pain behind his breastbone accompanied with frequent belching. After going to sleep, some nights he wakes up with a sore throat and a sour taste in his mouth. When questioned about his lifestyle, the physician found that most of George's daily food consumption occurred during hastily consumed evening meals. He jogged two or three miles per day several times a week.

The physician recommended several lifestyle changes for George. He began a new pattern of three evenly spaced meals per day. He was told to decrease his intake of fatty and spicy foods. George elevated the head of his bed to minimize reflux while lying down. Finally, the physician instructed George to take over-the-counter antacids when symptoms occur.

George followed up with his doctor a few months later and was able to report that his reflux symptoms had greatly diminished and were now under control.

51. In summary, should lifestyle modifications be implemented to reduce GERD symptoms?

It is apparent from this discussion on lifestyle modifications that the benefits obtained are mixed. Physicians are likely to recommend lifestyle modifications as a first step to alleviate GERD symptoms, since there are few if any adverse side effects from its adoption and there can be many benefits from lifestyle modifications in addition to GERD relief. Due to the many variables involved, the results of lifestyle modifications need to be evaluated on a case-by-case basis.

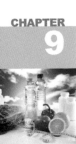

CHAPTER

9

What drugs and medications make GERD worse?

52. What are the reasons some drugs and medications used to treat conditions other than GERD can make GERD worse?

Certain medications can contribute to GERD in three ways (Thompson 2009):

- Medications can relax the LES allowing increased reflux to occur. Medications can either affect the nerves controlling the LES or the muscles that that control the tension of the LES.
- Medications can irritate and directly damage the esophagus increasing inflammation already caused by reflux.
- Medications can slow down digestion allowing food to remain in the stomach and causing an increase in acid production.

53. How can medications exacerbate GERD?

The internal organs of the body, such as the stomach, LES, esophagus, blood vessels, and the windpipe contain smooth muscle. These muscles are controlled by nerves of the autonomic nervous system in order to perform essential functions necessary for living. Medications used to treat certain conditions result in relaxation of smooth muscle. Since the LES is smooth muscle, it is also relaxed.

The autonomic nervous system controls body functions that are largely subconscious or involuntary. Digestion is an example.

DEFINITION

54. What medications can cause or exacerbate reflux (Humphries 1999, Go 2003)?

- *Anticholinergic medications*: These medications block the action of the autonomic nerves. These medications are commonly used to treat nausea by slowing digestion. By inhibiting nerve impulses to the LES, they relax the LES. Examples of antinausea medications include prochlorperazine (Compazine), promethazine

(Phenergan), and scopolamine
(Transderm Scop).

Examples of medications are presented as "generic name (Trade name)"—for example, "diazepram (Valium)." It should be noted that the following is not a comprehensive listing of medications, but simply contains some examples.

- *Asthma medications*: Asthma attacks result in contraction of airway smooth muscle. Drugs called *beta2-adrenergic receptor agonists* relax smooth muscle resulting in *bronchodilation*, or opening of the bronchi in the lung. The drugs also cause relaxation of the LES. An example of a bronchodilator is theophylline (Uniphyl, Theo-Dur).
- *Sedatives or tranquilizers*: When the actions of these medications depend on muscle relaxation, they will also relax the LES. Examples of drugs of these drugs include diazepram (Valium) and temazepam (Restoril).
- *Antidepressants*: Many medications used for depression affect the autonomic nervous system. Examples include amitriptyline (Elavil), doxepin (Sinequan), and imipramine (Tofranil).
- *Estrogen replacements*: As mentioned previously, estrogen in the body may be directly associated with GERD. Estrogen replacements are commonly used by post-menopausal women.

55. What medications directly irritate the esophageal lining?

- *Bisphosphonates:* These drugs are used to treat osteoporosis and can directly irritate the esophagus. When taking the pills, the patient is advised to drink plenty of water and to not lie down for a period of time. These measures are designed to wash the drugs through the esophagus as soon as possible. Examples of bisphosphonates include alendronate (Fosamax), ibandronate (Boniva), and risedronate (Actonel).
- *Non-steroidal anti-inflammatory drugs (NSAIDs):* These drugs are commonly used to alleviate headache or to reduce inflammation. They can irritate both the esophagus and stomach. Examples include aspirin, ibuprofen (Motrin, Advil), and naproxen (Aleve).
- *Antibiotics:* Certain antibiotics can also irritate the esophagus and stomach. Examples include erythromycin,

tetracycline (Sumycin, Tetracyn), Doxycycline (Vibramycin), clindamycin (Cleocin), and trimethoprim sulfa (Bactrim, Septra).

- *Potassium supplements:* Slow-release potassium chloride tablets like K-Dur can also irritate the esophageal lining.

56. What medications promote GERD by slowing digestion?

- *Blood pressure medications:* Calcium-channel blockers and beta blockers act on the smooth muscles of blood vessels, dilating them, and reducing blood pressure. The medications also delay stomach emptying and reduce tension of the LES. Examples of calcium channel blockers include felodipine (Plendil), diltiazem (Cardizem), and nifedipine (Procardia). Examples of beta blockers include metoprolol (Toprol), atenolol (Tenormin), and bisprolol (Zebeta).
- *Narcotics* are used for pain suppression, but they also slow digestion. Examples of narcotics include morphine (Avinza, Duramorph), ocycodone (Oxycontin), and fentanyl (Sublimaze).

57. How can I minimize the adverse effects of certain medications?

If you have GERD, and it is necessary to treat your other medical conditions, it is essential to consult with your doctor or pharmacist about all your medications. When medications have the potential to exasperate GERD, several steps can be taken:

- Alternative medications that are less detrimental to GERD may be available.
- Medications that irritate the stomach should be taken while sitting or standing up and with plenty of water. This will help wash the medications promptly out of the esophagus.
- Medications may be available with a protective coating so that they do not dissolve in the esophagus.
- The timing of taking supplements can be important. Taking the medications after meals or on an empty stomach could minimize damage.
- Taking ginger supplements or tea may minimize symptoms.

References

CHAPTER 7

1 Festi, Davide, Eleonora Scaioli, Fabio Baldi, Amanda Vestito, Francesca Pasqui, Anna Rita Di Biase, and Antonio Colecchia. "Body weight, lifestyle, dietary habits, and gastroesophageal reflux disease." *World Journal of Gastroenterology* 15, no. 14 (April 14 2009): 1690–1701.

2 Jones, Roger, Harley R. Liker, Philippe Ducrotté. "Relationship between symptoms, subjective well-being and medication use in gastro-oesophageal reflux disease." *International Journal of Clinical Practice* 61, no. 8 (2007): 1301–7.

3 Kaltenbach, Tonya, Seth Crockett, and Lauren B. Gerson. "Are Lifestyle Measures Effective in Patients with Gastroesophageal Reflux Disease?" *Archives of Internal Medicine* 166, no. 9 (2006): 965-71.

4 Lagergren, Jesper. "Influence of Obesity on the Risk of Esophageal Disorders." *Nature Reviews Gastroenterology and Hepatology* 8 (2011): 340–7.

5 Mayer, Emeran A. "The neurobiology of stress and gastrointestinal disease." *Gut* 47 (2000): 861-869.

6 Mittal, Ravinder K., Hubert A. Shaffer, Stella Parollisi, and Lane Baggett. "Influence of breathing pattern on the esophagogastric junction pressure and esophageal transit." *American Journal of Physiology* 269, no. 4 Part 1 (1995): G577–G583.

7 Mizyed, Ibraheem. "Review article: Gastro-oesophageal Reflux Disease and Paychological Comorbidity." *Alimentary Pharmacology & Therapeutics* 29, no. 4 (2009): 351–8.

8 NY Times Health. "Anxiety - In-Depth Report." *The New York Times.* January 30, 2013.

CHAPTER 8

9 Festi, Davide, Eleonora Scaioli, Fabio Baldi, Amanda Vestito, Francesca Pasqui, Anna Rita Di Biase, and Antonio Colecchia. "Body weight, lifestyle, dietary habits, and gastroesophageal reflux disease." *World Journal of Gastroenterology* 15, no. 14 (April 14 2009): 1690–1701.

10 Griffin R. Morgan. "Foods That Fight Heartburn." WebMD (2013). http://www.webmd.com/digestive-disorders/features/foods-that-fight-heartburn

11 Johnson Thomas Eugene, Lauren B Gerson, Tiberiu Hershcovici, Christopher Stave and Ronnie Fass. "Systematic review: the effects of carbonated beverages on gastro-oesophageal reflux disease." *Alimentary Pharmacology & Therapeutics* 31, no. 6 (2010): 607-14.

12 Kaltenbach, Tonya, Seth Crockett, and Lauren B. Gerson. "Are Lifestyle Measures Effective in Patients with Gastroesophageal Reflux Disease?" *Archives of Internal Medicine* 166, no. 9 (2006):965-71.

13 Meining Alexander, and Meinhard Classen. "The Role of Diet and Lifestyle Measures in the Pathogenesis and Treatment of Gastroesophageal Reflux Disease." *American Journal of Gastroenterology* 95, no. 10 (2000): 2962-7.

14 Nilsson, Magnus, Roar Johnsen, Weimin Ye, Kristian Hveem, and Jesper Lagergren. "Obesity and Estrogen as Risk Factors for Gastroesophageal Reflux Symptoms." *Journal of the American Medical Association* 290, no. 1 (2003): 66-72.

15 Talalwah, Narmeen. "Gastro-oesophageal reflux. Part 1: smoking and alcohol reduction." *British Journal of Nursing* 22, no. 3 (2013): 140-142, 144-146.

CHAPTER 9

REFERENCE

16 Go, Mae. "Medications That Exacerbate GERD." *Medscape Family Medicine*, August 27, 2003. http://www.medscape.com/viewarticle/460311

17 Humphries T.J., and G.J. Merritt. "Review article: drug interactions with agents used to treat acid-related diseases." Alimentary Pharmacology & Therapeutics 13, Suppl. 3 (1999): 18-26.

18 Thompson, Dennis. "Medications Linked to GERD." Everyday Health (2009). http://www.everydayhealth.com/gerd/treating-gerd/medications-that-worsen-reflux.aspx

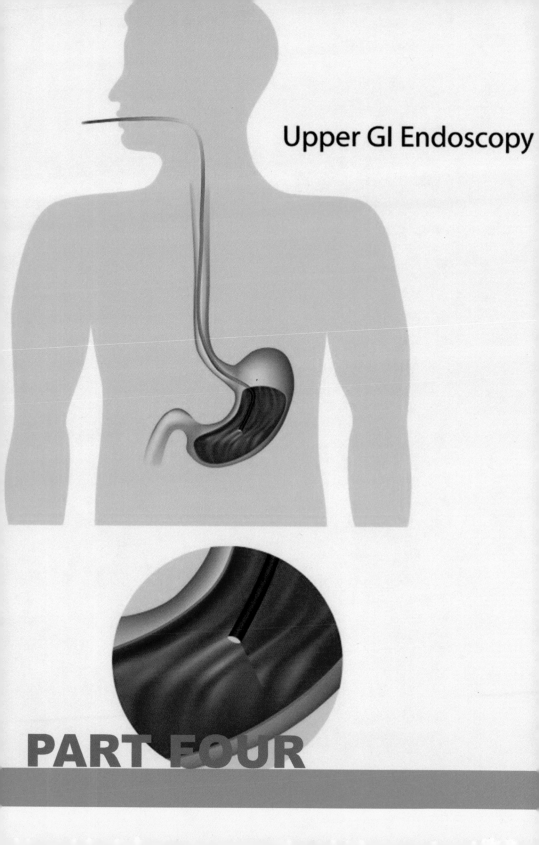

Upper GI Endoscopy

PART FOUR

Diagnosing and Treating GERD

In Part Four, we begin by discussing the tests used to diagnose GERD. We then discuss the medications used to treat GERD. Finally, when medications cannot control GERD, various surgical options are considered.

Diagnosing GERD

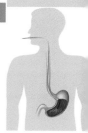

58. What is the first step in diagnosing GERD?

People typically self-treat symptoms of heartburn and regurgitation with the use of antacids. People may self-treat for months or even years before consulting a doctor, especially if the symptoms seem to be under control. When symptoms begin to affect the person's well-being, a primary care physician should be consulted. When the symptoms appear uncomplicated, the doctor may make a provisional diagnosis of GERD. The doctor may recommend some lifestyle changes, and may prescribe a more specialized GERD medication, such as a proton pump inhibitor or a H2 blocker.

If the symptoms are more complicated, the physician may refer you to a gastroenterologist, a specialist in diseases of the digestive tract. The specialist may order one or more tests to determine the cause or causes of the symptoms; it may be GERD, another gastrointestinal disease, or multiple causes.

59. What is a barium study?

An upper GI series is also known as a barium study or barium esophagram. An upper GI series can help diagnose the cause of abdominal pain, nausea and vomiting, swallowing problems, and unexplained weight loss. The test could reveal inflammation or swelling of the GI tract, scars or strictures, ulcers, hiatal hernia, and abnormal growths (NDDIC 2014). Many of these conditions are associated with GERD or its complications.

The procedure uses a liquid suspension of barium that coats the inner surfaces of the pharynx and esophagus allowing the surfaces to be better visualized on standard x-rays. The procedure could also use a procedure called fluoroscopy, which is a study of moving body parts. A continuous x-ray beam is passed throughout the body part being examined and the resulting images transmitted to a monitor, allowing the dynamics of esophageal motion to be visualized.

To ensure the upper GI tract is clear, health care providers usually advise people not to eat, drink, smoke, or chew gum during the 8 hours before the procedure. An x-ray technician and a radiologist—a doctor who specializes in medical imaging—perform an upper GI series at a hospital or an outpatient center.

A person does not need anesthesia. The procedure usually takes about two hours to complete.

For the test:

- the person stands or sits in front of an x-ray machine and drinks a barium salt.
- the person lies on the x-ray table and the radiologist watches the barium move through the GI tract on a monitor.
- the technician may press on the abdomen or ask the person to change positions to fully coat the upper GI tract with the barium.

After an upper GI series, a person can expect the following:

- bloating or nausea for a short time after the procedure
- to resume most normal activities after leaving the hospital or outpatient center
- barium in the GI tract that causes stools to be white or light colored for several days after the procedure

The radiologist will interpret the images and send a report of the findings to the person's gastroenterologist.

The risks of an upper GI series include:

- constipation from the barium—the most common complication of an upper GI series.
- an allergic reaction to the barium or flavoring in the barium.
- bowel obstruction—partial or complete blockage of the small or large intestine. Although rare, bowel obstruction can be a life-threatening condition that requires emergency medical treatment.
- a very small risk of cancer due to radiation exposure

60. What is an upper endoscopy exam?

For a doctor's eye view of an upper endoscopy exam look at a YouTube video:

https://www.youtube.com/watch?v=8V6VsNkGfTQ

ON THE WEB

An **upper endoscopy test** is often performed when a barium study does not provide enough details for a diagnosis. An endoscopy test is appropriate to determine the causes of GERD-related symptoms such as swallowing problems, nausea and vomiting, and abdominal pain. Examination of the esophageal interior can detect constrictions or rings, hiatal hernia, precancerous cells, inflammation or swelling, and ulcers.

Preparation work is necessary before the test. The patient cannot eat or drink after midnight the night before the test. Any medications that could affect bleeding must be forgone a few days before the test, and the patient is advised not to drive or work during the day of the test.

The procedure uses an **endoscope**, which is a narrow flexible tube of fiber optic cables with a video camera at one end. An external light source brings in light to illuminate the interior of the GI tract being examined. As the physician navigates the endoscope through the GI tract, electronic signals are transmitted up the scope to a computer which then displays the image on a large video screen.

A sedative is administered before the test, and the doctor usually sprays the throat to numb it. The doctor then inserts the endoscope down the throat, and passes the endoscope through the many bends of the GI tract. Digital images of key findings can be recorded.

An open channel in the endoscope allows other instruments to be passed through in order to take tissue samples. The samples are then viewed with a microscope to look for abnormalities that may be caused by acid reflux. If there is narrowing of the esophagus, it can be treated or dilated at this time. Esophageal dilation will be discussed under Surgical Procedures.

The endoscopy test is an outpatient procedure that requires only a brief recovery time for the effects of the sedative to wear off. Your throat may be a little sore, and you might feel bloated because of air introduced into the stomach during the procedure.

Complications are rare. Bleeding may occur at a biopsy site or where a polyp was removed. **Perforation** (a hole or tear) in the GI tract is very uncommon.

61. What is esophageal dilation?

Esophageal dilation can be performed at the same time as endoscopy. The procedure allows your doctor to dilate, or stretch, a narrowed area of your esophagus (ASGE 2014). GERD patients may have narrowing of the esophagus as a result of inflammation and scarring from acid reflux. Narrowing may also be due to esophageal rings or webs, cancerous tumors, or esophageal motility disorder.

At times, there may be uncertainty as to whether your symptoms may be due to GERD. The symptoms may atypical, or you may have tried GERD medications that have not alleviated the symptoms. These situations may prompt your physician to conduct a pH study.

A pH study measures when and how much acid enters into your esophagus. The doctor inserts a small tube that acts as a probe up the nose and down into the esophagus. The probe is attached to an **event recorder** that measures the amount of acid in the esophagus for 24 to 48 hours while you go about your normal activities. The doctor may require you to keep a diary to record when, what, and how much food you eat. The doctor may be able to see correlations between symptoms and reflux episodes.

The strength of acids are determined by their H+ ion concentrations; the greater the H+ ion concentration, the stronger the acid. H+ ions are also known as protons as they are hydrogen atoms that have lost their electrons. *pH* is a measure of the concentration of H+ ions in the liquid environment of the digestive tract. A pH of 7 is neutral, pH values of less than 7 are acid, while pH values above 7 are basic (alkaline). Stomach acid is strong hydrochloric acid with a pH ranging from 2–4.

NOTE

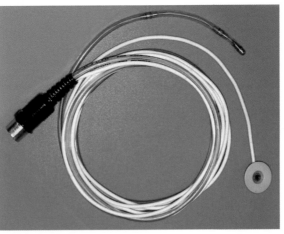

◀ **FIGURE 10.1**
pH probe for measuring acidity in the gastrointestinal tract

63. When would a manometry study be useful?

A **manometry** or **motility study** may be ordered by a physician to further diagnose **dysphagia** (difficulty in swallowing), or **odynophagia** (pain when swallowing) when an endoscopy test is normal. A manometry study measures the functioning of the esophagus and the LES by means of pressures generated during swallowing of food and liquids.

As mentioned, peristalsis is a complex process and involves the coordination of the upper esophageal sphincter, the esophagus, and the LES. During swallowing, the upper esophageal sphincter must open to allow the food bolus to enter the esophagus, peristalsis must propel the bolus toward the LES, and the LES must open to allow the bolus to enter the stomach. Achalasia is an uncommon condition that occurs when the LES does not open properly; it is often associated with faulty peristalsis. Diffuse esophageal spasm is another rare condition characterized by poorly coordinated contractions of esophageal muscle. Esophageal manometry may be recommended if you are considering surgery for GERD, since surgery will not cure conditions of achalasia or spasms.

The study uses a catheter attached to several pressure sensors. To conduct the study, a physician anesthetizes a patient's nose and guides the catheter through the nose into the stomach. The catheter is slowly withdrawn while the patient is asked at times to swallow either nothing or sips of water. Various pressure readings are taken in the stomach or throughout the esophagus. The pressure readings are analyzed to evaluate functioning of the esophagus and sphincters.

GERD Medications

64. What is the overall strategy for treating GERD by medications?

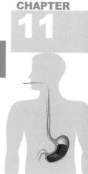

Three classes of medications are commonly used for treating GERD: antacids, H2 blockers, and proton pump inhibitors. Baclofen and prokinetic agents are also occasionally used. Treatment usually begins with the use of antacids to alleviate symptoms of mild heartburn or indigestion. Antacids are inexpensive, available over-the-counter, rapid acting, and with few side effects. If symptoms of GERD persist or if complications arise, it is necessary to turn to more effective and specialized medications; H2 blockers and proton pump inhibitors.

65. What are antacids and how do they work?

For a YouTube video on "How do antacids work?" visit:

https://www.youtube.com/watch?v=EXGHpXlBgZA

ON THE WEB

Antacids are bases which react with stomach acids by a process of neutralization, resulting in a reduction of stomach acidity. The goal of antacid use is to reduce **excess** stomach acidity, since acid is still needed for digestion. Antacids also inhibit the action of the digestive enzyme pepsin, since pepsin only works in an acid environment.

66. When should antacids be used?

All antacid products are available **over-the-counter** (OTC) without a doctor's prescription. Antacids are commonly the first medications used to treat mild symptoms of indigestion or heartburn. They are noted for being quick-acting but are of short duration. Antacids are effective for about three hours when taken after meals, since the food in the stomach slows down the emptying of stomach contents into the duodenum. If antacids are taken before meals, the antacids may provide acid reduction for only 20 to 40 minutes. Antacids should be used for only brief or intermittent periods, but if symptoms persist, or are of a serious nature, other medications should be used.

67. What are antacids composed of? (Monson 2013)

Antacid medications contain salts of sodium, calcium, magnesium, or aluminum, singly or in combination. Different formulations have been developed that vary in onset of neutralizing action, neutralizing capacity (the amount of acid a given amount of antacid can neutralize), and duration of neutralizing action. The choice of antacid may be based on the need for fast relief of acid reflux or for long lasting relief. Some antacids have additional ingredients to help the effectiveness of the medication.

Simeticone is an antifoaming agent that helps to reduce the gas (and pressure) in the stomach. The reduced pressure helps maintain the LES closed, resulting in less reflux. Products containing simeticone include Maalox Anti-Gas® or Mylanta Gas®.

Alginates have been used in some antacid formulations, particularly Gaviscon®, for over 30 years. Alginates are formulated with sodium or potassium bicarbonates and may contain calcium and magnesium salts as well. When alginates encounter stomach acid, they form a gel. The acid breaks down the bicarbonate into carbon dioxide gas which becomes entrapped within the gel converting it into foam. The foam floats on the surface of the gastric contents like a raft on water thus giving rise to the common name, "alginate rafts." (Mandell 2000) Alginates may bind to the esophageal mucosa and serve as a protective barrier between the esophagus and refluxate. Antacids with alginates have an additional advantage of providing longer-lasting relief, up to four hours.

68. What are some examples of antacids?

a. **Sodium antacids** contain sodium bicarbonate. They are potent and fast-acting but of short duration. They are commonly dissolved in water resulting in effervescence. Examples are Alka-Seltzer® and Bromo-Seltzer®. People on a low sodium diet may want to avoid using sodium-containing antacids.

b. **Calcium antacids** contain either calcium carbonate or calcium phosphate. Examples are Tums®, Alka-2®, and Titralac™. Calcium antacids have longer duration of neutralizing action.

c. **Magnesium salts** come in many forms. Magnesium salts have a mild laxative effect and can cause diarrhea. Examples are Maalox®, Riopan®, Gelusil®, and Mylanta®. Magnesium antacids have a short duration of neutralizing action.

d. **Aluminum salts** come as the hydroxide, carbonate gel, or phosphate gel. Aluminum salts have a long duration of neutralizing action. Since aluminum salts can cause constipation, they are often combined with magnesium salts to balance digestive action. Combination aluminum-magnesium antacids have an intermediate duration of action. Examples are Rolaids®, AlternaGEL®, and Amphojel®.

69. Can antacids interact with other medications?

Antacids are usually innocuous, especially when used only infrequently. Just like other medications, however, antacid use can cause adverse side effects. The potential for antacid-drug interactions is dependent on the chemistry and physical properties of the antacid preparation (Sadowski 1994). Since antacids change gastric pH, they may alter drug effects in the body by modifying the extent of drug dissolution, breakdown, or absorption from the digestive tract (Ogawa 2011). If you are taking other medications it would be best to consult with your doctor or pharmacist to determine if there could be adverse drug interactions with antacids. Also, certain medical conditions make it particularly risky to take antacids. These conditions include high blood pressure, heart disease, and chronic kidney disease.

When antacids are taken with acidic drugs, they can decrease the absorption of the drugs from the digestive tract, causing lowered blood levels of the drugs. As a result, the effectiveness of the drugs can be reduced.

Antacids can increase the absorption of drugs such as pseudoephedrine or levodopa resulting in possible toxic effects due to increased blood levels of the drugs.

Sodium bicarbonate increases the acidity of the urine, which can affect the excretion of some drugs by the kidneys. Thus, sodium bicarbonate increases the excretion of acidic drugs, and inhibits the excretion of basic drugs.

Antacids will continue to be used to treat mild conditions of acid reflux, but have been largely replaced by more effective drugs for serious symptoms of GERD.

70. When antacids do not work, what is the next step in medications?

For a brief introduction to H2 blockers and proton pump inhibitors, see the following YouTube video:

ON THE WEB

https://www.youtube.com/watch?v=vmkdZxl0hGI

Antacids work by neutralizing stomach acids already present but they provide only short-term relief. H2 blockers and proton pump inhibitors are known as **antisecretory medicines,** as they reduce or block acid production. Studies have shown that the likelihood of curing esophagitis is directly related to a medication's antisecretory effect (Kahrilas 2008).

71. How do H2 blockers work?

Histamine is a common organic compound in the body with many functions, including stimulating gastric acid production. Histamine is synthesized in gastric glands located in the mucosa of the stomach. Histamine is released from the glands by stimulation from nerves and gastrin hormone, which in turn are stimulated by the processes of food intake, food in the stomach and stomach distension. Histamine binds to H2 receptors located on the parietal cells in the stomach epithelium, stimulating the cells to produce acid. Histamine antagonists work by blocking the receptor and thereby preventing histamine from stimulating the acid-producing cells. H2 blockers are also known as histamine type 2 receptor antagonists (H2RAs). H2 blockers reduce stomach acid production, while PPIs totally block acid production. Tolerance to H2 blockers generally develops within two weeks of repeated administration, resulting in a decline in acid suppression.

72. Should you take H2 blockers?

H2 blockers were the mainstay of treatment for GERD in the 1980s. They are available as OTC medications and in stronger dosages as prescriptions. H2 blockers can be effective in reducing symptoms of mild or moderate acid reflux and in treating inflammation of the esophagus. H2 blockers are now used much less frequently than before due to the arrival of the more effective proton pump inhibitors.

There are four H2 blockers available by prescription: cimetidine (Tagamet®), ranitidine (Zantac®), nizatidine (Axid®), and famotidine (Pepsid®). They are considered to be equally effective.

73. How should you take H2 blockers?

H2 blockers come in a variety of formulations: capsules, pills, chewable, liquid, or effervescent.

OTC dose preparations containing half of the lowest prescription dose are sold in small amounts for short-term use. The OTC preparations are typically taken twice daily, while prescription doses are typically given once daily at bedtime (Thompson 2009). OTC H2 blockers may be used for up to two weeks for short-term symptom relief, while prescription H2 blockers may be used on a long-term basis to relieve persistent GERD symptoms.

74. What are the side effects from using H2 blockers?

Since H2 blockers act primarily in the stomach, the major side effects involve the stomach and digestion. These side effects occur in about 5% of patients, and include constipation, diarrhea, nausea, and vomiting.

75. What are proton-pump inhibitors and how do they work?

While H2 blockers act by preventing histamine from stimulating acid production in the parietal cells, **proton-pump inhibitors** (PPIs) block the enzyme system responsible for secreting H+ ions into the lumen of the stomach. PPIs, therefore, block the last stage of gastric acid secretion. The PPIs are given in an inactive form (Wikipedia 2014). The PPIs cross the parietal cell membranes to bind with and inactivate the proton-pump enzyme system. As we mentioned, protons are H^+ ions, which are characteristic of acids.

76. What are examples of proton-pump inhibitors?

Proton-pump inhibitors should be used only when antacids fail to improve symptoms or resolve complications of acid reflux. PPIs have been used for over 25 years, and have largely supplanted H2 blockers due to their superior effectiveness. All PPIs appear to be similarly effective.

Examples of PPIs available over-the-counter (OTC) are: omeprazole (Prilosec®OTC and Zegerid®OTC) and lansoprazole (Prevacid®24 HR).

Examples of PPIs available by prescription include: esomeprazole (Nexium®), Prilosec®, Prevacid®, rabeprazole (Aciphex®), dexlansoprazole (Dexilant®), Zegerid®, and pantprazole (Protonix®).

77. How should you take PPIs?

PPIs control GERD by preventing acid secretion. PPIs need one to two days to start working, so are of little value to take after symptoms of acid reflux are occurring.

OTC PPIs have potencies of about one-half the prescription potencies for the same drugs. OTCs are only intended for short-term

(14 day) courses of treatment for up to 3 times a year. If OTC use does not resolve reflux symptoms, a doctor should be consulted. The doctor may then order a prescription dose.

It is best to establish a schedule of taking PPIs around 30 to 45 minutes before meals. Given the chronic nature of GERD, PPIs may need to be taken on a regular basis and not sporadically.

CASE STUDY

Jim was experiencing symptoms of acid reflux for the last six months, consisting of burning behind the breastbone and an occasional acidic taste in his month. He used antacids, but found they only relieved symptoms temporarily. When his symptoms began to occur daily and started to disturb his sleep, he decided to consult his physician. The physician decided the symptoms were very typical for GERD, so further testing was not necessary. Since PPIs are usually more effective than histamine-2 receptor antagonists for patients experiencing moderate reflux symptoms, the physician prescribed generic omeprazole. After four weeks on the medication, Jim returned to his physician to report a complete relief of symptoms. (CADTH 2007)

78. What are the side effects of PPI medications?

Similar to H2 blockers, the most common side effects from using PPIs include diarrhea, nausea, and vomiting. Diarrhea is a greater problem with PPI use, occurring in about 5–10% of patients.

Other serious complications can occur from PPI use, particularly in people susceptible to certain conditions. These complications, described in the following paragraphs, are rare.

PPIs (as well as other antacid preparations) lead to an elevated risk developing food allergies by suppressing the acid-mediated breakdown of proteins. These undigested proteins then pass into the small intestine, potentially leading to sensitization to a range of foods or drugs. It is unclear whether this risk occurs with only long-term use or with short-term use as well (Pali-Scholl 2011).

Studies have shown that patients receiving PPIs have a greater risk of acquiring pneumonia either in their community or in the hospital. The association between H2 receptor antagonist use and pneumonia risk is less strong. The decreased secretion of gastric acid may allow bacterial overgrowth in the digestive tract which is subsequently drawn into the lungs by aspiration. The acid-suppressing drugs may also encourage bacterial growth in the respiratory tract by inhibiting an enzyme (Chun-Sick Eom 2011).

The Food & Drug Administration (FDA) has revised its "Drug Facts" labels on prescription PPI medications to reflect possible increased risk of fractures of the hip, wrist, and spine with the use of the medications. The FDA acknowledges that the greatest risk is for people who take prescription medications for over one year or who have been taking high doses of the prescription medications. The FDA recognized that the risk of fractures for people taking OTC PPIs according to label directions is unlikely (FDA 2012).

The FDA issued a warning that omeprazole can reduce the effectiveness of the blood clot lowering drug clopidogrel (Plavix©) when both drugs are used simultaneously (AHRQ 2011). This publication also gives comparative prices of GERD medicines (as of 2011).

79. When is baclofen used to treat GERD?

Baclofen (trade names Lioresal, Gablofen) is related to **gamma-aminobutyric acid** (GABA), a naturally occurring neurotransmitter. Neurotransmitters are chemicals that nerves use to communicate with one another. GABAB receptors are proteins located on the surface of neurons (nerve cells). GABA binds to the receptors, stimulating a biological process resulting in inhibition of nerve impulses that would cause LES relaxations (such as during stomach distension). Since baclofen is similar in structure to GABA, it also binds to and activates the receptors, resulting in an enhanced inhibitory effect (Wise 2004).

Baclofen was developed as a treatment for spastic movement disorders, and is also used in topical creams as a muscle relaxant. Baclofen has also found limited application in treating GERD. The drug acts to prevent reflux by reducing transient LES relaxations rather than by blocking acid production. Baclofen's mode of action is therefore attractive to some practitioners since it focuses on blocking **all** reflux components, acid as well as non-acid.

Baclofen tends to be used when PPIs are not totally effective in treating GERD, or when they become refractory (lose their effect). Baclofen can be used together with PPIs, or by itself. Although baclofen is known to cause drowsiness, this has not apparently been a problem when used in treating GERD.

80. What are prokinetic agents?

Prokinetic (promotility) agents enhance the strength and coordination of muscular contractions in the stomach and small intestine, thereby enhancing the emptying of the stomach. These drugs also strengthen the LES.

The first prokinetic drug, Cisapride, appeared on the market in the early 1980s, and proved very effective in treating GI motility disorders, including gastropareisis (stomach paralysis), severe constipation, chronic intestinal pseudo-obstruction, and GERD. Unfortunately, due to severe side effects such as irregular heartbeat, it was removed from the market.

Prokinetics currently on the market include bethanechol (Urecholine), and metoclopramide (Reglan). These drugs also have serious side effects.

Currently, prokinetics are generally used only in serious cases of GERD, when other medications are ineffective. They can be used singly or in combination with other GERD medications. Reviews of the literature indicate that using prokinetic drugs may improve GERD symptoms in patients, but have little benefit on esophageal healing (Manzotti M 2007, Ren 2014) Prokinetics are also used in certain cases of GI motility disorders.

Surgical Procedures

CHAPTER 12

81. When should you consider surgery for your GERD?

Surgery is considered to be the final option for treating GERD when lifestyle changes and medications do not provide resolution of symptoms or do not heal lesions.

Medications (primarily PPIs) have many advantages and a few disadvantages for treating GERD:

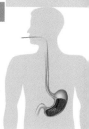

Advantages:

- Easy to use tablets taken orally
- Non-invasive compared to surgery
- Very effective on relieving symptoms and healing lesions of GERD
- Adverse side effects of PPI use are rare
- Relatively inexpensive, especially if used short-term

Disadvantages:

- Does not correct the underlying causes of GERD
- Continuous maintenance therapy frequently required to prevent recurrence of the disease
- Symptoms persist in at least 10% of patients
- May not correct complications of GERD

Surgery also has advantages and disadvantages that need to be carefully considered:

Advantages:

- Strengthens the LED, thereby controls reflux, the underlying cause of GERD
- Very effective in improving quality of life
- Generally eliminates the need to take GERD medications post-operatively
- Patients receive the psychological benefit of not having to cope with chronic disease
- May provide effective treatment of GERD complications, such as upper respiratory tract symptoms that are difficult to treat medically.
- Provides means of curing GERD in particular groups of people with certain genetic and congenital abnormalities

Disadvantages will be discussed in detail in the section on Nissen fundoplication. The following listing is a summary:

- Invasive method, but less so with laparoscopic technique
- Risk of postoperative complaints, such as dysphasia
- Rare but potentially severe postoperative complications

82. What is laparoscopic surgery and how has it benefited GERD treatment?

Laparoscopy is a minimally invasive type of surgery that involves less risk and fewer complications than conventional surgery. Patients who have laparoscopic surgery generally experience less pain and scarring after surgery, have a quicker recovery, and less risk of infection than those who have conventional surgery. Laparoscopic surgery has found broad application to treat many medical conditions, including GERD, and has also been used as a diagnostic tool.

Conventional GERD surgery involves using a scalpel to open a six-inch vertical incision in the abdomen. During laparoscopy, five or six small incisions are made in the abdomen. Then, the abdominal cavity is inflated with carbon dioxide to lift the abdominal wall away from the organs below and provide an operating space in the abdomen.

The laparoscope and surgical instruments are inserted through the incisions. The surgeon is guided by the laparoscope, which transmits a picture of the abdomen on a video monitor so the procedure can be performed.

83. What is Nissen fundoplication?

Nissen fundoplication was developed as a conventional surgery to treat GERD. **Fundoplication** means folding of the fundus. The procedure is now preferably done laparoscopically, unless the patient has a large hiatal hernia or other major complications of GERD. The surgery is not usually performed on older people, especially if they have other medical problems. The surgery would not be performed if the patient has an esophageal peristalsis disorder.

Before starting the surgery, the surgeon inspects the abdomen to make sure the surgery will be safe to perform. The presence of scar tissue, infection, or unsuspected abdominal disease would be reasons not to perform the surgery.

If hiatal hernia is present, the surgeon will return the herniated stomach back to the abdominal cavity, repair the hiatus, and wrap a portion of the fundus around the LES (Figure 12.1). In the

ON THE WEB

For an excellent 55-minute webcast on Nissen fundoplication surgery, go to:

http://www.orlive.com/shawneemission/videos/watch-a-live-surgical-webcast-for-treatment-of-acid-reflux?view=displayPageNLM

This webcast was prepared in 2009, when the Nissen procedure was state-of-the-art. In addition to a close-up visualization of the surgery, the surgeons make extended commentary on GERD topics that we have been discussing.

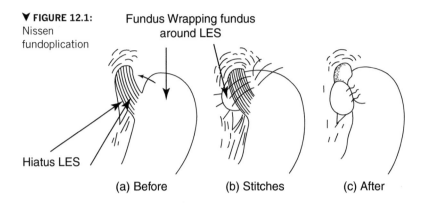

▼ FIGURE 12.1: Nissen fundoplication

Fundus Wrapping fundus around LES

Hiatus LES

(a) Before   (b) Stitches   (c) After

NIH IMAGES: http://search.usa.gov/search/images?affiliate=nih&cr=true&page=1&query=nissen+fundoplication

A. Total (Nissen)   B. Partial (Toupet)

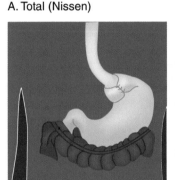
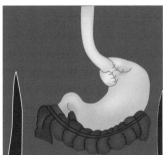

◀ FIGURE 12.2 Total & partial fundoplication

SOURCE: Treatment Options for GERD or Acid Reflux Disease—A Review of the Research for Adults,
AHRQ Publication 11-EHC049-A
Agency for Healthcare Research and Quality
U.S. Department of Health & Human Services

Nissen fundoplication procedure, the fundus is totally wrapped around the LES (Figure 12.2a), while in a modification called the Toupet procedure, the fundus only partially encircles (270°) the LES (Figure 12.2b). The purpose of the wrapping is to reinforce and strengthen the LES to facilitate its closing against reflux. There is some indication that patients who undergo the Toupet procedure experience less dysphagia while maintaining reflux control, compared to patients who undergo the Nissen procedure (Zornig 2002).

84. What are the complications from fundoplication procedures?

When skilled surgeons perform the operation, immediate post-surgical complications are rare. These complications can include perforation of the esophagus or stomach, injury to the spleen, and pneumothorax (collapsed lung). Common to many surgeries, patients may experience nausea (Richter 2013). It is very important to perform a successful surgery the first time, as a repeat surgery is more likely to result in complications and is less likely to resolve the reflux problem. Most failures occur within the first two years of the initial operation.

Surgical failures can involve tissue movements after surgery, including the following:

- A hiatal hernia may occur in which both the gastroesophageal junction and the surgical fundus wrap move through the hiatus into the chest.
- A hiatal hernia may occur in which only the gastroesophageal junction passes through the hiatus.
- A paraesophageal hernia may occur.

The purpose of the surgery is to strengthen the LES to minimize transient LES relaxations. However, if the surgery makes the LES too tight to open when necessary, it can lead to complications. These complications are:

- Inability of the food bolus to pass into the stomach, leading to dysphasia. Patients with dysphasia are treated with dietary modification that usually resolves the condition within 2-3 months.
- A group of complaints known as **gas-bloat syndrome resulting** from the inability to vent gas from the stomach after fundoplication. These symptoms can include bloating, abdominal distension, early satiety, nausea, flatulence, inability to belch, and inability to vomit.
- Atypical symptoms of GERD recur, including lung, ear, nose, throat, and chest pain involvement.

Fortunately, most problems with dysphagia or gas-bloat syndrome resolve during the first year after surgery.

85. Why are endoscopic procedures performed?

Patients with GERD are reluctant to undergo surgery (even the less invasive laparoscopic method) due to the perceived post-surgery complications. Several less invasive endoscopic procedures have been developed that can be just as effective as surgery in treating GERD. The patient's gastroenterologist will determine if the patient is a good candidate for an endoscopic procedure.

86. What is transorial incisionless fundoplication?

Transorial incisionless fundoplication (TIF) is an endoscopic procedure that uses a patented device called **EsophyX** to repair and reconstruct the LES. The TIF procedure can be suitable under most conditions where anatomical correction (surgery) is necessary. TIF differs from traditional fundoplication procedures because it is performed through the mouth rather than through laparoscopy or open abdominal incisions.

During the procedure, EsophyX is inserted in the patient's mouth together with the endoscope, and passed through the LES to the beginning of the fundus. The endoscope illuminates the surgical site while the EsophyX picks up a portion of the fundus lining and folds it adjacent to and partially encircling the LES. During the procedure, small hiatal hernias (two centimeters or less) can also be treated by stretching the esophagus. The fold is stitched in place where it heals naturally.

The TIF procedure can be an attractive surgical alternative for patients that have GERD symptoms unsatisfactorily controlled by PPI medications. Studies have shown that patients undergoing TIF report a significant improvement in GERD symptoms and a significant discontinuation of PPI use. (Trad 2012, Testoni 2010). The TIF procedure does not result in an overly tight fundoplication, so that problems of dysphasia and gas bloat are minimized.

For an interesting video on the TIF procedure, visit:

ON THE WEB

http://www.gerdhelp.com/about-tif/

Risks associated with the procedure are usually temporary, and can include sore throat, shoulder pain, dysphasia, nausea, or vomiting.

87. How is the radiofrequency ablation procedure used to treat Barrett's esophagus?

Ablation is the removal of biological tissue. Prior to the procedure, patients with high-grade dysplasia undergo an endoscopic ultrasound procedure to ensure that the dysplasia has not spread to deeper tissues. The radiofrequency ablation procedure itself is endoscopic and is performed on an outpatient basis. The device used in the procedure is an electrode mounted on an endoscope. The patient is anesthetized and the endoscope is inserted into the esophagus to the location of the Barrett's esophagus. Heat energy is delivered directly to the diseased lining resulting in destruction of the tissue. The tissue sloughs off over a period of 48 to 72 hours after the procedure. An attractive aspect of the procedure is that over a period of six to eight weeks, the tissue is replaced by normal (squamous) lining (Shaheen 2009, Frantz D2010).

Following the procedure, patients are placed on a modified diet to allow time for the tissue to heal. Of course, patients will continue on a rigorous schedule of GERD medications. About 20% of patients will experience chest pain following the procedure, and a small number may develop esophageal stricture requiring dilations.

ON THE WEB

To view a short video on the radiofrequency ablation procedure, visit:

http://www.mayoclinic.org/ diseases-conditions/barretts-esophagus/multimedia/ radiofrequency-ablation/ vid-20084711

88. What is a Stretta procedure?

The Stretta procedure also uses radiofrequency energy, but is applied to the LES instead of the esophagus. Although the mechanism of action is uncertain, radiofrequency heat energy applied to the LES may cause contraction and thickening of the muscle tissues with a deposition of collagen. Collagen fibers are commonly found in the body to provide strength and elasticity to tissues.

The radiofrequency procedure was described in the previous Question. In Stretta, the overlying mucosa is protected from damage by irrigation of the site with cooled sterile water to maintain the temperature below 50°C (Franciosa 2013).

Following the procedure, patients are instructed to take liquids for 24 hours, followed by a soft diet for one week. Patients continue taking anti-reflux medications for at least three weeks, and then gradually reduce medications as GERD symptoms improve.

Overall, patients are satisfied with the results of surgery, reporting a large decrease in anti-reflux medication use, and improvement in quality of life.

89. What patients could benefit from a Stretta procedure?

Ideal patients for the Stretta procedure should have GERD symptoms that are not satisfactorily controlled with PPI therapy, who have pathologic acid reflux, and have low grade esophagitis.

Patients who are not good candidates for the procedure have a hiatal hernia larger than 2 cm, have Barrett's esophagus, have significant dysphasia, have high-grade esophagitis, or have inadequate peristalsis. If the patients do not fit these criteria, they may be offered a fundoplication procedure (Richards 2003).

90. Should you consider endoscopic surgery?

Endoscopic devices were developed in the early 2000s to treat GERD by TIF or radiofrequency energy. Since that time multiple studies have demonstrated the safety and effectiveness of the procedures, and they have become mainstream procedures at many medical centers.

References

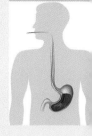

CHAPTER 10

1   National Digestive Diseases Information Clearinghouse "Upper GI Series." Publication No. 14-4335. (May 7, 2014). http://digestive.niddk.nih.gov/ddiseases/pubs/uppergi/

2   American Society for Gastrointestinal Endoscopy. "Understanding Esophageal Dilation." 2014. http://www.asge.org/patients/patients.aspx?id=392

CHAPTER 11

3   Agency for Healthcare Research and Quality. 2011. "Treatment Options for GERD or Acid Reflux Disease-A Review of the Research for Adults." AHRQ Pub. No. EHC049-A.

4   CADTH (2007). Physicians' Interactive Education Case Studies, Canadian Agency for Drugs and Technologies in Health.

5   Eom, Chun-Sick, Christie Y. Jeon, Ju-Won Lim, Eun-Geol Cho, Sang Min Park, and Kang-Sook Lee."Use of acid-suppressive drugs and risk of pneumonia: a systematic review and meta-analysis." *Canadian Medical Association Journal* 183, no. 3 (2011): 310-9.

6   Food and Drug Administration "Possible Increased Risk of Bone Fractures With Certain Antacid Drugs." *Consumer Health Information* (2012, May 2010). http://www.fda.gov/downloads/ForConsumers/ConsumerUpdates/UCM213307.pdf

7   Kahrilas, Peter. "Gastroesophageal Reflux Disease." *New England Journal of Medicine* 359, no. 16 (October 2008): 1700-7.

8   Mandel K.G., B. P. Daggy, D. A. Brodie, and H. I. Jacoby. "Review article: alginate-raft formulations in the treatment of heartburn and acid reflux." *Alimentary Pharmacology & Therapeutics* 14 (2000): 669-90.

9   Manzotti, Matías, Hugo N Catalano, Fernando A. Serrano, Gisela Di Stilio, María F Koch, and Gordon Guyatt. "Prokinetic drug utility in the treatment of gastroesophageal reflux esophagitis: a systematic review of randomized controlled trials." *Open Medicine* 1, no. 3 (2007):E 171-80.

10 Monson, Kristi. "Antacids." MedTV (2013). http://gerd.emedtv.com/antacids/antacids.html

11 Ogawa Ryuichi, and Hirotoshi Echizen. "Clinically significant drug interactions with antacids: an update." *Drugs* 71, no. 14 (October 1 2011): 1839-64.

12 Pali-Schöll, Isabella, and Erika Jensen-Jarolim. "Anti-acid medication as a risk factor for food allergy." *Allergy* 66, no. 4 (2011): 469-77.

13   Ren, Li-Hua, Wei-Xu Chen, Li-Juan Qian, Shuo Li, Min Gu and Rui-Hua Shi. "Addition of prokinetics to PPI therapy in gastroesophageal reflux disease: A meta-analysis." *World Journal of Gastroenterology* 20, no. 9 (2014): 2412-2419.

14   Sadowski, Daniel C. "Drug interactions with antacids. Mechanisms and clinical significance." *Drug Safety: an international journal of medical toxicology and drug experience* 11, no. 6 (1994): 395-407.

15   Thompson, W. Grant. "H2 Blockers-Indications, Effectiveness and Long-term Use." International Foundation for Functional Gastrointestinal Disorders. Publication 528-GERD (2009).

16   Wikipedia (2014). "Proton-pump inhibitor", Wikipedia, the free encyclopedia. http://en.wikipedia.org/wiki/Proton-pump_inhibitor

17   Wise, James and Jeffrey Conklin. "Gastroesophageal reflux disease and baclofen: is there a light at the end of the tunnel? *Current Gastroenterology Reports* 6, no.3 (June 2004):213-9.

CHAPTER 12

REFERENCE

18   Effective Health Care Program/Agency for Healthcare Research and Quality. "Treatment Options for GERD or Acid Reflux Disease: A Review of The Research for Adults." AHRQ Publication No. 11-EHC049-A (September 2011). http://www.effectivehealthcare.ahrq.gov/ehc/products/165/756/gerd_consumer.pdf

19   Franciosa, Mark, George Triadafilopoulos, and Hiroshi Mashimo. "Stretta Radiofrequency Treatment for GERD: A Safe and Effective Modality." *Gastroenterology Research and Practice* (2013), Article ID 783815, 8 pages.

20   Frantz, David J., Evan S. Dellon, and Nicholas J. Shaheen. "Radiofrequency ablation of Barrett's esophagus." *Techniques in Gastrointestinal Endoscopy* 12, no. 2 (April 2010):100–7.

21   Richards, William O., Hugh L. Houston, Alfonso Torquati, Leena Khaitan, Michael D. Holzman, and Kenneth W. Sharp. "Paradigm Shift in the Management of Gastroesophageal Reflux Disease." *Annals of Surgery* 237, no. 5 (May 2003): 638–49.

22   Richter, Joel. Gastroesophageal Reflux Disease Treatment: Side Effects and Complications of Fundoplication." *Clinical Gastroenterology and Hepatology* 11, no. 5 (May 2013):465–71.

23   Shaheen Nicholas J., Prateek Sharma, Bergein F. Overholt, Herbert C. Wolfsen, Richard E. Sampliner, Kenneth K. Wang, Joseph A. Galanko, Mary P. Bronner, John R. Goldblum, Ana E. Bennett, Blair A. Jobe, Glenn M. Eisen, M. Brian Fennerty, John G. Hunter, David E. Fleischer, Virender K. Sharma, Robert H. Hawes, Brenda J. Hoffman, Richard I. Rothstein, Stuart R. Gordon, Hiroshi Mashimo, Kenneth J. Chang, V. Raman Muthusamy, Steven A. Edmundowicz, Stuart J. Spechler, Ali A. Siddiqui,

Rhonda F. Souza, Anthony Infantolino, Gary W. Falk, Michael B. Kimmey, Ryan D. Madanick, Amitabh Chak, and Charles J. Lightdale. "Radiofrequency Ablation in Barrett's Esophagus with Dysplasia." *New England Journal of Medicine* 360 (2009): 2277-88.

24 Testoni Pier A., Maura Corsetti, Salvatore Di Pietro, Antonio Gianluca Castellaneta, Cristian Vailati, Enzo Masci, and Sandro Passaretti. "Effect of Transoral Incisionless Fundoplication on Symptoms, PPI Use, and pH-Impedance Refluxes of GERD Patients." *World Journal of Surgery* 34, no. 4 (April 2010): 750–7.

25 Trad, Karim S., Daniel G. Turgeon, and Emir Deljkich. "Long-term outcomes after transoral incisionless fundoplication in patients with GERD and LPR symptoms." *Surgical Endoscopy* 26, no. 3 (Mar 2012): 650–60.

26 Zornig, Carsten, Ursula Strate, Christiane Fibbe, Alice Emmermann, and Peter Layer. "Nissen vs Toupet laparoscopic fundoplication." *Surgical Endoscopy* 16, no. 5 (May 2002): 758–66.

Index

GERD symptoms
    exercise, 38–39
    foods and beverages on, 40–45
    obesity, 37–38
    smoking, 38
    stress, 39–40

H

H2 blockers
    formulation, 61–62
    PPIs (*see* Proton-pump
      inhibitors)
    prescribed, 61
    side effects, 62
    working, 61
H. pylori infection, 17
Heart attack. *See* Chest pain
Heartburn, 17, 18. *See* Acid reflux
Hiatal hernia, 15–16
Hiatus, 13, 14, 16, 67, 69
Histamine, 61
Histamine type 2 receptor
    antagonists (H2RAs), 61
H2RAs. *See* Histamine type 2
    receptor antagonists

I

Indigestion. *See* Dyspepsia
Inner mucosal layer, 10
Internal sphincter, 13
Irritable esophagus, 24

L

Laparoscopy, 66–67
Laryngitis, 28
Laryngopharyngeal reflux (LPR),
    28
Larynx, 9–10
LES. *See* Lower esophageal
    sphincter
Lifestyle modifications, 45
Lower esophageal sphincter (LES),
    12
    lower pressure of, 15
    transient relaxations, 15

M

Magnesium salts, 59
Manometry, 56–57
Medications
    advantages and disadvantages,
      65–66
    antacids, 58–60
    baclofen, 64–65
    contribution of, 46
    esophageal lining, irritation in
      antibiotics, 47–48
      biophosphonates, 47
      NSAIDs (*see* Non-steroidal
        anti-inflammatory drugs
        (NSAIDs))
      potassium chloride, 48
    exacerbate GERD, 46
      anticholinergic medications, 46
      antidepressants, 47
      asthma medications, 47
      estrogen replacements, 47
      sedatives or tranquilizers, 47
    H2 blockers, 61–62
    H2RAs (*see* Histamine type 2
      receptor antagonists)
    minimizing adverse effect of, 48
    PPIs (*see* Proton-pump
      inhibitors)
    prokinetic agents, 65
    promoting GERD, by slow
      digestion
      blood pressure medications, 48
      narcotics, 48
Motility study. *See* Manometry
Muscularis, 11

N

Narcotics, 48
Nasopharynx, 29
Nissen fundoplication, 67–68
    complications, 69
Non-acid reflux, 4, 30–31
Non-steroidal anti-inflammatory
    drugs (NSAIDs), 47
Non-ulcer dyspepsia, 20

Nose, 29–30
NSAIDs. *See* Non-steroidal anti-inflammatory drugs
Nutcracker esophagus, 23

O

Obesity, 37–38
Odynophagia, 56
Over-the-counter (OTC), 58

P

Paraesophageal hiatal hernia, 15, 16, 69
Peptic stricture. *See* Esophageal stricture
Peptic ulcers, 17
Perforation, 55
Peristaltic action, 14
pH study, 56
Pharynx, 9
Pleurisy/Pleuritis, 18
Pneumothorax, 18–19
Potassium chloride, 48
PPIs. *See* Proton-pump inhibitors
Prevalence
    adults, 5
    among women and men, 4–5
    children, 5
    overall, 4
Prokinetic agents, 65
Proton-pump inhibitors (PPIs)
    definition and working, 62
    examples of, 62
    procedure for taking, 62–63
    side effects of, 63–64
Pulmonary embolism, 18
Pyloric valve, 14

R

Radiofrequency ablation, 71
Radiologist, 53
Regurgitation, 19–20
Rolling type, hiatal hernia, 15

S

Saliva, 9, 20, 29
Sedatives /tranquilizers, 47

Simeticone, 58
Sinuses, 30–31
Sliding type, hiatal hernia, 15
Smoking, 38
Sodium antacids, 59
Squamous cell carcinoma, 27
Steakhouse syndrome, 24
Stress, 39–40
Stretta procedure, 71–72
Submucosa, 11
Surgical procedures
    advantages and disadvantages, 66
    endoscopic procedures, 70, 72
    laparoscopy, 66–67
    nissen fundoplication, 67–68
    radiofrequency ablation, 71
    stretta procedure, 71–72
    TIF (*see* Transorial incisionless fundoplication)
    toupet procedure, 68
Symptoms, GERD, 4, 17–21
    chest pain, 18
    dyspepsia, 20–21
    heartburn, 17, 18
    regurgitation, 19–20

T

Teeth, injury, 29
TIF. *See* Transorial incisionless fundoplication
Toupet procedure, 68
Trachea, 9–10
Transient LES relaxation, 13
Transorial incisionless fundoplication (TIF), 70

U

Upper endoscopy test, 53–54
Upper GI series. *See* Barium study

X

X-ray technician, 53